I0797430

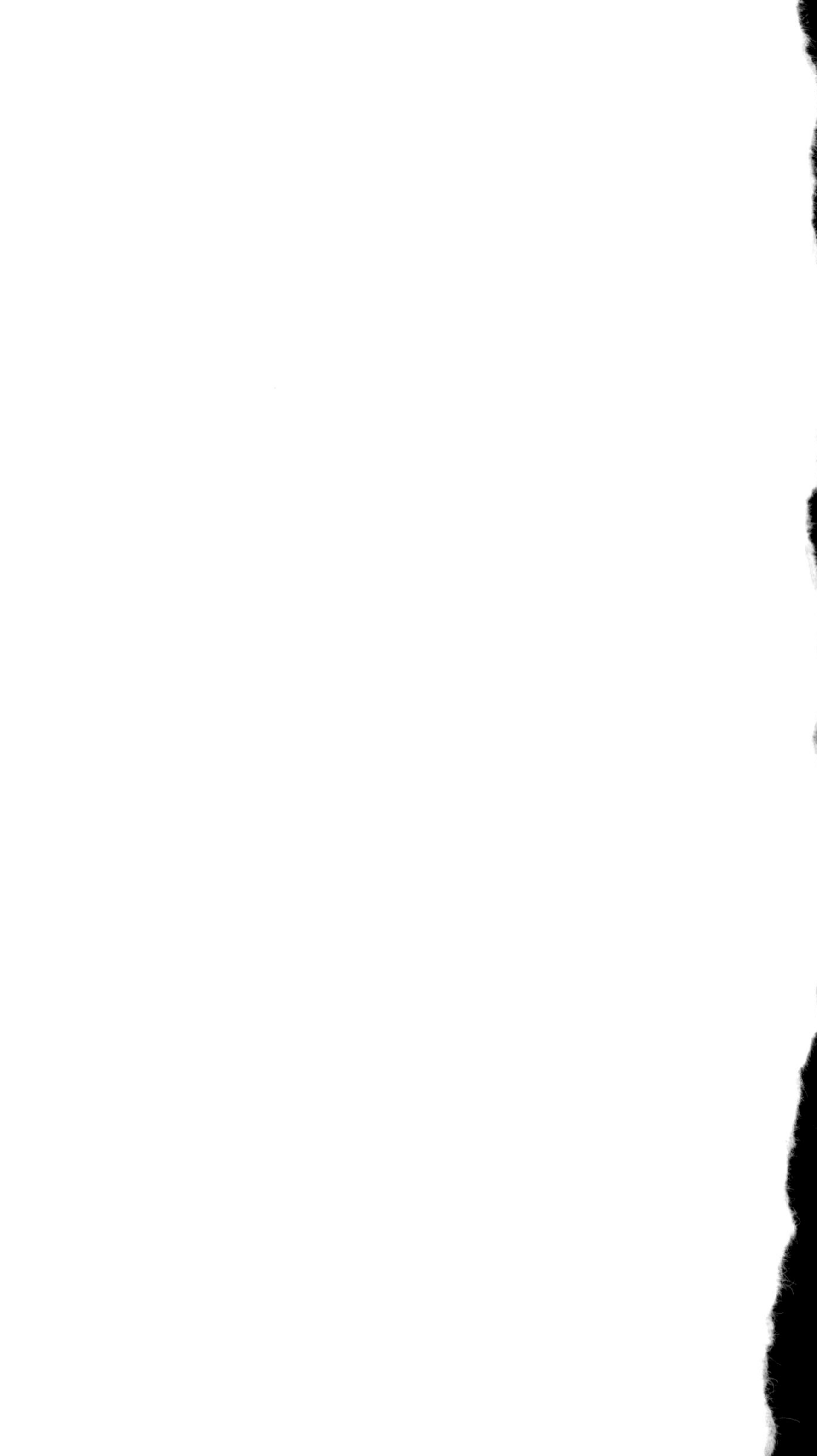

TOUGH ENOUGH

TOUGH ENOUGH

HONE YOUR HABITS,
CULTIVATE PURPOSE,
AND FORGE
GENUINE STRENGTH

TREY TUCKER

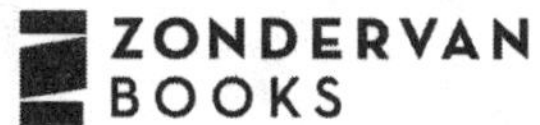

ZONDERVAN BOOKS

Tough Enough

Published by Zondervan, 3950 Sparks Drive SE, Suite 101, Grand Rapids, MI 49546, USA. Zondervan is a registered trademark of The Zondervan Corporation, L.L.C., a wholly owned subsidiary of HarperCollins Christian Publishing, Inc.

Requests for information should be addressed to customercare@harpercollins.com.

Zondervan titles may be purchased in bulk for educational, business, fundraising, or sales promotional use. For information, please email SpecialMarkets@Zondervan.com.

ISBN 978-0-310-37056-7 (hardcover)
ISBN 978-0-310-37285-1 (South Africa edition)
ISBN 978-0-310-37058-1 (audio)
ISBN 978-0-310-37057-4 (ebook)

HarperCollins Publishers, Macken House, 39/40 Mayor Street Upper, Dublin 1, D01 C9W8, Ireland (https://www.harpercollins.com)

Cover design: Micah Kandros
Cover illustration: Shutterstock
Interior design: Kristina Juodenas

Printed in the United States of America

25 26 27 28 29 LBC 5 4 3 2 1

A MAN WHO LACKS PURPOSE DISTRACTS HIMSELF WITH PLEASURE.

VIKTOR FRANKL, PSYCHOLOGIST AND PHILOSOPHER

AUTHOR NOTE

This is a work of nonfiction, based on research and professional insight. All case studies are real, but in most cases, names, identifying characteristics, and circumstances of people described in the book have been changed to protect identity. I've done my best to be faithful to experiences so that shared lessons are most helpful.

CONTENTS

INTRODUCTION

You can become the man you were meant to be—the man you quietly yearn to be.

And I'm here to help you get there.

As a licensed mental health therapist, I work with young men every day—men who are smart, capable, and full of potential, yet still feel stuck. I've listened closely. I've seen the patterns. I've walked beside them as they faced the hard stuff—and found their way forward.

Maybe you're battling anxiety or depression. Maybe you constantly feel like you're not enough. Maybe you've been chasing money, sex, or substances, hoping they'll fix what's missing—but they never do. Maybe you've started to believe there's no way out, that you're stuck with these feelings—and the regret and shame that come with them.

But you're not stuck. You're stronger than you know. And it's time to move forward.

You weren't made to drift through life distracted, numb, or angry. You were made to thrive—fully awake, fully alive, and deeply grounded in the genuine strength of who you are. You have it in you to become the kind of man who doesn't chase approval or hollow pleasure but who builds a life of purpose instead. A man who leads with quiet confidence. A man who knows how to navigate setbacks. A man who loves boldly, stands tall, and fights for something—not because he must, but because he chooses to.

You don't have to fake being tough. You simply must learn how to get tough enough to meet life head-on and thrive.

In this book, you'll learn how to do that and more:

- **how to cut out distractions** that have kept you stuck—whether it's the noise of the world or the lies you've believed about yourself
- **how to build your team**—the people who make you better and won't let you quit
- **how to identify and heal hidden injuries** that are quietly shaping your life
- **how to unleash the anxiety assassin**—a mindset shift that helps you stop anxiety before it controls you
- **how to harness your inner caveman**—your drive, your grit, your raw power—not to suppress it, but to focus and channel it

This journey isn't about perfection; it's about learning to stop running—from your fears, from your past, from yourself—and choosing to grow instead. Because the world doesn't need more fake toughness. It needs you—a man of real strength who is tough enough to become all you are meant to be.

1

YOU ARE NOT A PUPPET (TAKE ACTION TO KILL DISTRACTION)

Distraction is the enemy of everything you're capable of becoming.

It steals your time, energy, attention—your potential. But here's the good news: I see young men fight back against distraction and win all the time. You can too. You can take back control if you are willing to step back, get honest about where your focus is taking you, and make the most of your time and attention.

First, understand this: You are not alone. Struggling with

distraction doesn't mean you're lazy or undisciplined; it means you haven't yet seen how deeply it's impacting your life or learned how to fight it.

We all battle distraction at one level or another. But for many young men today, it's more than a nuisance; it's an epidemic—a silent one that quietly undermines your confidence, your relationships, your mental health, and your future. But it doesn't have to. You have the power to change your trajectory—starting now. And I'm here to help you and others like you.

That's why I'm sitting in my office, biting my tongue so I don't bark and scare off the young man in front of me. I want to help. I ask him a question, but he doesn't respond. His eyes are locked on his iPhone, fingers tapping, swiping. I'm not even sure he heard me.

I gently ask him to put his phone away. He slips it into his pocket and turns his gaze out the window.

That's what distraction does.

It disconnects us from each other—and from ourselves.

And if we don't deal with it, it wins—keeping our life off course.

Wes is twenty-two, a senior in college, and he's made an appointment with me, a licensed therapist who specializes in helping young men find their confidence, whole-body strength, and true manhood. I help them improve mental health without wasting time on the fluff. Men like Wes come to me because they want a direct, straight-to-the-point approach to mental health. They want to skip the flowery language that sometimes accompanies counseling and dig to the root of the issue.

That's when they tap into life-changing growth and transformation and find their true strength.

Wes has everything he thought he wanted when he began college nearly four years earlier—a circle of friends, a girlfriend, and the academic transcript he'd need to get a good-paying job.

About a month ago, he even finished his biggest project as a college student, leading a concentrated effort in his fraternity to help provide food for students on strict budgets. On paper, he's checking all the boxes for good to go. And he doesn't show any warning signs of substance misuse or substantial mental health trouble of any kind.

But it isn't always a major problem that sets us back.

Small problems can become big problems when ignored.

That's where I come in, helping Wes and other young men address what keeps them from optimizing their lives and flourishing in all aspects, including lifting up those around them—family, friends, and community. My job is to help Wes find and cultivate his focus so he can become the man he wants to be.

What Wes is going through is what many, perhaps even most, men in my practice experience: They know they aren't where they want to be—where they need to be—but they aren't sure what the problem is or how to solve it. What I do in my work, and what this book is about, is helping men see clearly and get to where they want to be.

The problem for Wes is that despite the work he's done to position himself for success, he feels like he's drowning as graduation approaches. He says he is not overwhelmed by anything specific, but by everything at once.

As Wes looks out the window, he tells me he didn't want to see me. The appointment was his girlfriend's idea—her demand, in fact, he explains. She told him he'd seemed flat and generally frustrated for weeks—agitated by simple conversations and unhappy, battling malaise, not wanting to do things he typically enjoyed.

"She also said I'm drinking and smoking too much," Wes said, rolling his eyes.

"Is she important in your life?"

"Yeah, I mean, sure. I'd like to marry her once I get settled in a job."

I ask Wes how often he drinks alcohol to excess or smokes, and he says in quick response, "Not much, I mean, not like some of my friends."

I ask him to define how often is not much, and Wes says that recently his alcohol consumption has increased to several binges a week of four or more drinks, and that typically he and friends smoke while drinking, often leading to hangover and next-day agitation as the substances wear off.

But "it's my senior year," he says. "My last moments with college friends."

In my business as a therapist, we call Wes's response a contextual excuse, an attempt to justify behavior that is harming that person's life and relationships.

We make such excuses due to fear, shame, guilt, or uncertainty, and they keep us from doing what we should do or want to do but don't do. In other words, the excuses make an easy way out of tough situations we don't want to face, even if we want a better outcome.

The excuse is our rationalization.

Wes says he wants to marry his girlfriend in the future, but she says his behavior is about to chase her away. Yet he keeps doing it anyway.

"What else am I supposed to do my senior year?" Wes asks, as if he's preparing for a final exam on drinking and smoking.

The problem, Wes explains, is that when he and his girlfriend met his freshman year, he barely drank at all and never used marijuana, focusing instead on establishing himself in college as a solid student. Now, he says, she doesn't want to move forward with their relationship beyond graduation if he doesn't figure out what's bothering him and stop the self-medicating and denial.

"It was seek counseling or else," Wes says.

So, here we are, me and Wes, who doesn't want to be here. It's going to be fifty minutes of extreme awkwardness if I can't get Wes to relax and take a deeper look at what's bothering him. That's why my first task is to earn his trust.

"Hey, man," I say. "Listen, I'm glad you're here. I understand that you probably don't want to be here. I get it. Your girlfriend. An ultimatum. But here we are, because you asked for the meeting. We have a little time, so let's talk."

If Wes suspects I'm pushing an agenda, I might as well be playing tug-of-war with a pit bull. In recent years, much of the stigma around counseling has dissipated, particularly for young men, helping them put down their armor during the work. Still, young men are often the hardest to get to talk or share their true inner struggles.

I get it, because I was once much the same way, puffing my chest to show strength and distract myself from what was really going on and from doing the harder work of looking inside. That's why I started my practice, Rugged Counseling, to meet young men where they are.

That's what I'm attempting with Wes.

"Let's not talk about your girlfriend right now," I say. "You made the appointment, so let me ask you: Are you happy with how you feel, with where your life is?"

Silence, as Wes turns his gaze out the window once again.

I let the silence burn.

"No," Wes says, eventually. "I'm not."

To make sure Wes knows he's in charge of where we go during our time together, I say, "Let's imagine we are sitting in a car. I'm in the passenger seat, and you are the driver. You're at the wheel. My role in the passenger seat is to point out some different streets we can go down, but you are always in charge. It's your decision which streets we travel on this trip together."

I can't assess what's wrong in Wes's life, or what got him here, without Wes revealing his truth. It's the same with you. It's the same for me. It's the same for everybody.

I must help a client like Wes figure out the direction to go rather than map it out for him because he holds the key to reclaiming his life and joy. I've told him he's safe with me, that I care about him, and that I'm listening, but he's at the wheel, in charge of where we go.

Wes smiles and looks me briefly in the eyes. I know that now we're getting somewhere.

For the next forty-five minutes, Wes takes me through a day in his life.

He says he wakes up, checks social media, and responds to

his likes and DMs so his friends won't think he's not engaged. All the while, he's texting with his girlfriend and talking with friends about plans for after classes and into the evening. Then he says he'll get a couple texts from his father, mother, and even his brother. They ask how his day is going and when he's coming home as if he didn't just talk to them.

Wes says he grabs a quick breakfast and gets to classes, managing more messages as he works on assignments during lunch. He says he typically goes to his friend's apartment after classes. They'll game for a couple of hours, drinking beer, smoking some weed, and munching on snacks until his girlfriend texts. She says he'll hurt her feelings if he doesn't stop by to see her, he explains. So he'll stop by for an hour. They talk and make out a little, but the whole time he's thinking about the classwork he needs to finish by tomorrow if he's going to get to the bar with his friend in the evening. He says he tells her he can't stay long. "Fine," she'll say, poking out her lip in disappointment.

Wes says usually before he knows it, he has stayed another hour and then he's off to the bar to meet his friend. They close it down because he figures he's only a senior once and he'll never get such an opportunity again.

Wes says he finally arrives home at 1:00 a.m., finding a snack in the refrigerator. Meanwhile, his girlfriend is texting him about the next day and he's scrolling through social media to make sure he hasn't missed anything. He'll finish the classwork blurry-eyed, get in bed at 2:00 a.m., and tell himself he'll watch a few TikTok videos to "relax a little" to get to sleep. Instead, he finds himself stuck watching one video after another, finally dozing off at about 3:00 a.m. The next morning, his alarm sounds at 7:30 a.m., and it's a repeat—a day in the life of a college senior who has it all together on paper.

But who is drowning.

When Wes finishes explaining his daily routine, I say with a chuckle, "That's it? That's all you do in a day?"

I let him think about what he's said. Distraction is a killer of success. For Wes. For me. For all of us. It takes and wastes so much of the time and energy we have for life.

Bestselling author Jon Gordon writes in his book *The Energy Bus* that "desire, vision, and focus" move your bus (life) in the right direction. "Remember," Gordon writes, "you have only one ride through life so give it all you got and enjoy the ride."[1]

Distraction keeps us from taking the ride in life we want.

Consider that research shows how distractions like social media, gaming, substance misuse, and pornography can even change our perceptions of what's real and what really matters.[2] Other impacts of distraction include:

- reduced attention and learning
- less focus on goals and others
- dissatisfaction
- increased stress and anxiety

Do you ever experience these feelings or issues? If so, distraction is likely your enemy.

When we're living in distraction, there's no room for faith. No space for growth. No foundation for sustained happiness—no joy. And that's where Wes is. He admits he's not happy. The girlfriend he wants to marry is threatening to leave. And yet he moves through the same damaging routine, like a puppet on strings—disconnected, distracted, and stuck.

"I feel guilty," Wes says, "and like a failure, even though I'm making good grades and about to graduate from college. I don't think I'm doing much at all, but I feel completely overwhelmed, like I can't organize or get ahead on anything."

BOREDOM IS A MESSENGER BEGGING YOU TO GROW

There's so much I could say to Wes from the beginning, like explaining the research that says time on electronic devices and social media before bed is an absolute deterrent to quality sleep—at any age.[3] Wes isn't alone in that, considering the average person spends two hours and twenty-four minutes on social media a day, a pace that would add up to seven years in an average lifespan.[4] We often call it entertainment, but more honestly, it is a practice of running from ourselves, feeding a constant need to distract from the present moment and anything we are facing or are needing to do. The same is true of substance misuse or friends who don't have our best interests in mind. We know it's not good for us, but we keep returning to doing it anyway because we haven't yet developed the recognition and tools that give us the strength to turn away.

Already I can see distraction is likely at the root of Wes's frustration, but he can't fix the problem until he's ready and able to see how and why he's distracted and then do something about it. I know this not only because I'm a professional, but because I have plenty of my own experience dealing with distraction, as do most men I counsel.

It's a common theme I'm increasingly seeing among the young men I work with. Like Wes, they've allowed distractions to take charge of their life, rendering them string puppets as opposed to men in control, men filled with purpose. The demands they experience are intense—from the pressure to be in constant contact with work, friends, and partners to the expectation of excelling in everything. It's enough to overwhelm anyone, and self-medication is a common response.

But the medication of distraction just leads to internal pressure building from everything ignored or diverted. It's like walking around with a soft drink bottle that's constantly shaken up. It needs a release, and if we don't do it properly, the result is what Wes is feeling—increasing anxiety, discomfort, and self-doubt.

The solution requires you to get tough enough to say no and work through your priorities, planning how you'll spend your time. It requires you to cut the puppet string to take charge of yourself rather than reacting like a marionette to external pulls, moving throughout the day without following your plan, which will leave you exhausted, frustrated, and joyless.

That's where Wes finds himself—as a puppet on a string.

On paper, everything in his life looks good. Grades—check. Girlfriend—check. Chances at a decent job at graduation—check. No obvious trouble. But inside he feels a churning he keeps trying to ignore, a churning that only comes back stronger the more he ignores it.

"I need it to stop," Wes says, opening up. "Not, like, I

need out of life. It's not that. I just need time to breathe and think. I feel awful the next day after drinking too much and giving myself and my girlfriend too little time. I don't want that. I feel numb racing through the days."

"What do you want?" I ask him.

Wes pauses.

"I want it to feel like I'm waking up for a reason, like, I've got a mission."

Now we're getting somewhere.

Wes is driving himself toward understanding, which leads to change. In one meeting, he identified the problem: He's overwhelmed and does not consider the activities he's spending time on valuable. Wes originally hadn't wanted to talk or pause to self-reflect, but now he's digging in—facing what he has been trying to ignore.

As with all of us, the more we try to avoid our unhappiness, the more unhappy we tend to become. And that's how it was for Wes. But once he faced and acknowledged the root problem, positive change began instantly.

"What do you see in your future?" I ask Wes.

"Possibility," he says, looking into my eyes, and I smile, because he has taken a big step toward becoming the man he wants to be.

Among the first things we must learn in addressing distraction is about the healing power of quiet. In the noise and distraction of daily life, our minds are reacting. We need quiet for thinking, for processing.

Studies show that time for silence restores the nervous system.[5] Useful practices for clearing our minds of anxiety involve creating moments of deep silence, especially in a natural environment.

It's easy to avoid deep silence in the busy world, with our phones lighting up with messages and so much coming at us. So much we want to do. I understand. I'm a go-getter, so long periods of quiet are not natural for me. But a couple years ago, I knew I needed to do something because something was off inside me.

The skies had been gray for a couple of weeks, and I wondered if that was what was wrong, that I'd come down with seasonal depression. Licensed therapists are like everyone else; we are not immune from seasonal depression, anxiety, or any other diagnosis in the mental health spectrum. Seasonal depression is a genuine diagnosis, affecting millions of Americans annually. It typically first appears in people's teenage years, and women are more affected than men, as are those living in regions including New England and Alaska. It wasn't something I had faced before and wasn't sure what I was experiencing was it. I felt more flat than depressed, and I knew that was common too.

We can sometimes get something milder than seasonal depression called the winter blues—not full-on depression, yet we aren't feeling the same joy from activities we usually enjoy. Not quite depressed, but easily distracted and bothered. That's where I was, not getting the most out of activities I usually enjoy, like lifting weights or going to concerts. I didn't know why.

I knew I needed to give my mind time to untangle and

process, but I realized I couldn't do that while just sitting still. I decided to combine light physical activity with time alone, but I'd make it hard—some rugged counseling for myself. In other words, I would put myself in an uncomfortable position of walking for hours away from distraction so I'd have to deal with the other uncomfortable burdens I was wrestling with, whatever they were.

I decided to walk for hours on nature trails at a national park without phone, music, or companion. Just me and the outdoors, walking, and learning about myself along the way. At first, feelings of frustration surfaced. Eventually, after a couple of hours, the source emerged: I craved companionship, someone special to experience life with, to make a family with, and I didn't have that.

There was no one to blame but myself. I'd fallen into the trap of a single life with short-term relationships when what I really wanted was something deeper, more lasting.

What I faced was no different from what Wes faced, except for the superficial circumstances. He kept returning to substance misuse and time distraction despite the fact that it was eroding his life and threatening to take away everything he wanted, including his relationship. I kept returning to the short-term relationships that were keeping me from finding the one thing I wanted.

Deep into my fourth hour of walking, I recognized that when I was younger, this behavior seemed to work, I suppose, in the sense that I got to meet many people. But it falsely stroked my ego and became a habit, like a powerful drug. I've never been drawn to alcohol or marijuana, but that doesn't mean I don't have issues. Most of us struggle with harmful habits of some kind, and for me, these brief encounters became addictive and costly—a short-term fix without long-term reward.

This realization was hard to face, even while walking alone on the trails of the park. It was embarrassing, and I felt myself cringe, step-by-step, with that self-admission. But each step got easier, and I felt my pace quicken, a burden lifted from my soul as I cried out in a prayer of hope and healing.

It's not uncommon to do things that actually go against what we want deep down. Like me, like Wes, our weaknesses and vulnerabilities will take us down roads of destruction if we allow them to. It's easy to fall into the trap of chasing short-term pleasure that can ultimately take away deeper joy and more lasting contentment. But just as we can lead ourselves into damaging situations, we are also the ones with the power to take ourselves out of them. That's why, even as I confronted a harsh truth, I was relieved, and I felt my blues drifting away because the first step to health is removing the distractions so we can better see ourselves.

When I got to my truck, I took several gulps of water and eagerly turned on my phone. Hours had passed since I feared unplugging. I wondered, *Did anyone truly need me?*

I smiled. I'd received only five messages and a couple of missed calls, none of them particularly urgent. The world had not missed me as much as my ego and my device addiction had assumed, and it turned out I hadn't missed the world or my phone much at all. I found more of myself on my walk, locked in without distraction, clearing my mind, and recentering my goals. I was eager to start enjoying life in the last days of winter as a better me.

What about you? Are you willing to create moments of deep silence? Are you willing to fight back against the many distractions life throws at you?

Odds are high that you are like Wes or me, even though the specifics may be different. Most of us are or will be distracted by something, or several somethings, that keeps us from where we want to go, from flourishing as joyful men. From sports betting to pornography to sex and smartphones and social media to alcohol and drugs, the addictive distractions that tempt men are many and challenging. And they are getting stronger each day, aiming to take us away from being the men we are called to be.

Because we're human, we're all at risk. But for young men, it's often more than that because we are more at risk for sports betting or gambling addiction, more prone to pornography addiction, and more likely to develop cannabis dependence or cannabis use disorder and alcohol use disorder.

Too often, I see young men struggling with some or all of these behaviors (or more) that began as distractions and then became unmanageable. With Wes, as with most clients, I got him to walk me through his daily life, which quickly revealed the many distractions he faced. You can easily audit your daily life and distractions by following this practice:

- Audit your time. Track several days, noting what you do, who you do it with, how much time you spend doing it, and how you feel afterward.

- Notice when you numb out.
- Ask yourself, *Did that time help me grow? Would I have felt better if I had spent time doing a different or healthier activity?*

With Wes, the turning point came when we did a time audit. It got his attention when he saw just how much of his day was lost to distractions. I encouraged him to take ownership of his time—starting with a simple plan.

The first step was identifying his goals. He listed things that mattered to him—spending more quality time with his girlfriend, having space to recharge, and focusing more effectively on school or work with less anxiety.

Wes built a daily plan that reflected those priorities. It started with a morning workout—which naturally made late-night drinking less appealing. He scheduled intentional time with his girlfriend. He reduced distractions by setting boundaries with his phone. And each evening, he set aside a few minutes for honest reflection: How did today go? Did I move closer to who I want to be? How do I feel about the day?

Within weeks, the change in Wes was visible. A broad smile returned to his face. His life had shifted—because he had taken control. Wes killed the distractions that were taking him down.

What's stealing your time and attention?

What's holding you back from becoming who you want to be?

You, too, can kill the distraction.

You, too, can reclaim your life.

TIPS

→ Right now, give your brain sixty seconds of silence. Just be still and let it rest.

→ Next, notice what your brain wanted you to do to escape the silence. If our brains aren't used to silence, they'll look for a way out of it because our brains crave what's familiar.

→ Tomorrow, increase this time to ninety seconds, then add thirty seconds each day.

2

RUN THROUGH DISCOMFORT

HE WHO IS NOT ANGRY, WHEREAS HE HAS CAUSE TO BE, SINS. FOR UNREASONABLE PATIENCE IS THE HOTBED OF MANY VICES, IT FOSTERS NEGLIGENCE, AND INCITES NOT ONLY THE WICKED BUT EVEN THE GOOD TO DO WRONG.

AUTHOR UNKNOWN, ***INCOMPLETE COMMENTARY ON MATTHEW***

Happiness and flourishing have little to do with having an easy life. If it did, we'd do little to nothing and be good with that. But that's not how it works.

Happiness and flourishing have to do with facing and conquering the obstacles and difficulties as it relates to where you are called to go and what you learn from failures and stumbles along the way. This may sound counterintuitive; culture lures us to chase the quick and easy and the feel good. But studies reveal that embracing discomfort can help us grow, which means that when we avoid discomfort, we don't grow.

Learning to face and run through discomfort is a core strength of a man. That's why it's important for us to work at cultivating toughness.

Don't like public speaking? Push yourself to do it and grow. Tend to avoid hard conversations that should be had? Push yourself to do it and grow. According to Kaitlin Woolley and Ayelet Fishbach, "Achieving personal growth often requires experiencing discomfort."[1]

Pushing ourselves is rarely fun at the beginning because the discomfort we fear usually comes immediately, trying to distract us and pull us up short. No one likes obstacles, and most of us, especially men, try to avoid discomfort.

That's why when something doesn't feel right or feels hard, our first instinct is often to run in the opposite direction. We take what seems like the easier path—not because it leads to something better, but because it feels less threatening in the moment. Even when, deep down, we know it'll make things harder for us later, we still tend to run away. In everyday life, it can look like this:

- men who skip doctor visits or ignore their health—putting their well-being at risk

- men who avoid opening up about what they're really struggling with—putting their relationships at risk
- men who cope with the pressure through hours of gaming, misuse of substances, or treating sex like a scoreboard—putting their futures, their jobs, and their sense of purpose at risk

Any of it, or all of it, puts our emotional health at risk, which then also makes life more difficult for the people in our lives, including friends, parents, coworkers, and significant others.

We can't avoid the little things, or the big things, and expect to win. We must face discomfort and manage it, or it will manage us.

A man who learns to face what lies before him not only alleviates discomfort but frequently preempts it. We need to channel our anger and impatience with discomfort in a way that enables us to face the discomfort head on so we can manage it rather than letting it scare us away.

Learning how to better understand ourselves—and how we can best *respond* rather than *react*—is vital, especially for men. Our egos and emotions can be fragile, no matter what we tell ourselves. And real toughness isn't about appearances or bravado; it's about inner strength—something we can learn, build, and grow over time—that comes from running through (not away from) discomfort.

Remember, everyone has a breaking point. But there is no limit to the resilience we can develop, which will take us almost anywhere we want to go. The key is learning how to run through the discomfort life throws at us—or we bring upon ourselves—so that we arrive healthier and stronger on the other side.

In small and large ways, I've been working on my approach to discomfort for as long as I can recall, and it has helped me better understand and appreciate areas in which I'm not as strong. Hand me a water bottle, and I'll twist off the cap with my left hand instead of my dominant right because doing so is harder and more uncomfortable. I'll take the stairs instead of the elevator, or I'll do the extra rep in the gym when I want to quit. Alternatively, I will call it a day even if my adrenaline says keep going; I know my body has done enough and I need to rest.

The little discomforts we move through prepare us for times when more significant challenges strike—like the time I took part in the fight against human trafficking and found myself in a dangerous situation in a foreign country.

On the surface, opening a bottle cap with my nondominant hand and fighting human trafficking have little in common, but they are, in fact, related. It's the cumulative effect of small things that yield big results. By practicing twisting bottle caps with my weaker hand or by always taking the stairs, I learned that I could do what my mind naturally wants to resist.

After watching the movie *Taken*, which is about an ex-CIA officer who tracks down two teenage girls kidnapped by human sex traffickers, I started researching the issue and learned that millions of people are trafficked for forced sexual exploitation.[2]

I discovered that dozens of nonprofit organizations worldwide were involved in the fight, but I knew I wanted to act, not just donate. I spent six months calling and emailing these organizations; most ignored me. They probably thought I was crazy for offering to help since I had no background in law enforcement.

The few that did respond said they had full-time, trained people who do this. But just as I was about to give up, one organization emailed me and said they were interested. I investigated them and they investigated me, and before long, I found myself on a team of five men between the ages of eighteen and fifty-five, traveling to a country in Asia with plans to take out a human trafficking ring.

I found myself in a country I'd never been to with four other men I'd never met, aiming to fight with little training a human crisis I had only recently learned about. Our mission was to find underage girls forced into sex work and free them from traffickers.

I was nervous and deeply uncomfortable. I had never been in a situation remotely like this one, and I had no confidence. Zero. I found myself in a strange city in a commercial strip lined with brothels, feeling so much sadness for the girls. But I pressed forward, letting my anger push me through my discomfort, because I wanted to stop the pimps, just like Bryan Mills in *Taken*.

As a therapist, I know what anxiety is, and I was in it. Full-throttle anxious. *What have I gotten myself into?* I wondered. This was extreme discomfort. I'd never felt that level of anxiety. For several nights leading up to the raid, I couldn't sleep. I found myself fixating on worst-case scenarios—catastrophizing, therapists call it, when someone exaggerates in their mind the potential negative outcomes of an impending situation. I reminded myself this was what I wanted—there was no backing down. In the end, we saved girls. A bar got shut down, traffickers got arrested, and underage girls received their freedom and crucial support.

This story is extreme, but the principle is the same for all of us. Because I had regularly practiced pushing through discomfort in many areas of my life, I had confidence that I could make it through anything and be all right.

The more we learn to face and run through discomfort, the more we will be able to face genuine and extreme adversity. Yes, I was in that situation by choice, but most of us will find ourselves in situations of stress or grief, facing circumstances that require us to push through hard and intense things we've never seen coming.

And when the big ones do come—like the death of a parent or a spouse, the loss of a job, or a relationship breakup, arriving at our doorstep as an unexpected and uninvited guest—we will discover the strength we have built by dealing with discomfort rather than wishing it away with avoidance.

That's why when my father died unexpectedly nearly a decade ago. I made myself deal with it rather than push the sadness away. He was my friend and mentor. Dad worked in education like me, as a longtime head of school, and he helped me understand the importance and value of working with young people. My father taught me that we can help shape young adults into who they are called to become, and we receive the same from them in return. That has been my calling. But then he died in a car wreck, and my friend and mentor was gone.

Knowing the importance of mourning and remembering

him as I processed his death, in the months after he died, I intentionally carved out thirty minutes a day to think about him, his life, and our life together. I did this so that the flood of thoughts wouldn't sneak up on me and take me by surprise. Some days, I'd write him a letter. On other days, I'd look through pictures or talk with him in my mind. Without a doubt, some days were painfully difficult because I felt his loss intensely. But by the end of each day, I always felt better.

Once we deal with what's uncomfortable, we feel better immediately and for the longer term. We become more confident, and with that confidence comes a virtuous cycle of less fear and anxiety, more resilience, and enhanced relationships.

PUTTING OFF UNTIL LATER IS THE ENEMY OF PROGRESS

The truth is that avoidance is easy, especially for common, ordinary things. Most of the discomfort we're tempted to avoid involves small day-to-day life issues. In my experience, this is particularly true of men in their twenties and thirties. And when small issues are ignored repeatedly, they grow in magnitude to become big problems.

That's about the time the men come to see me.

In a perfect world, these men would come sooner, before the problems take root. But, as the saying goes, better late than never.

Consider Miles, twenty-three, who was struggling at work with many tasks he doesn't enjoy. They had begun to overwhelm him, which led him to let them pile up.

As a senior in college the year before, Miles mostly chose what he wanted to do, except for a little studying, which didn't feel like work since he liked his major. He'd sleep late most days, play some basketball, work twenty hours a week at a part-time job, and watch hours of Netflix. With a B average and a job lined up in sales with a regional internet provider, Miles coasted into full-time work without giving any thought to his mental health.

Three-quarters of the year into his job, Miles had a good group of young professional friends and some friends from college he remained in contact with. The problem was with his job. He said he liked it initially, but after six months, he began to feel overwhelmed and uninterested in the onslaught of details—such as emails and reports—required to keep up. He said it kept piling up and most of it felt pointless. He started putting off tasks, telling himself he'd get to them later that day or the next. But when the next day came, much of the work was still left undone. Again.

More work came in, piling onto what he had ignored. By the time he arrived at my office to try to figure it out, the man who was a B student in college the year before, who liked his job initially, had fallen far behind at work, questioning his future. He was afraid he'd lose the job, but he also wanted to quit because he didn't know how to dig himself out.

Miles admitted he's a procrastinator in other areas. He'll ignore or put off household chores like doing the laundry, or he'll tell himself he'll exercise the next day but then he doesn't. He concluded by telling me he feels bad about himself for procrastinating.

I reminded him he's not the first to face this battle, and

then I asked, "Why do you think people avoid things, especially things they need to do?"

"I don't know," he said. "Maybe I'm lazy. That's what my dad says."

"That's an unfair statement to say about anyone, especially about yourself," I said. "There are always root causes underneath why people avoid tasks at work or home, or why they put off uncomfortable or unpleasurable things they need to do or want to do."

I paused, then said, "The desire to avoid discomfort is at the heart of all our procrastination. Not laziness. Avoidance has more in common with fear than laziness. So let me ask, What do you do with your time at work when you're avoiding these emails and reports?"

He paused.

"Online gambling," he said. "Mostly sports. I'm either reading about upcoming games to figure out how to bet on them, or if a game is underway, I'm making prop bets and general bets on the outcome."

"Do you win at gambling?"

"Not usually. No. But I go back to it anyway, ignoring the work I need to do."

"In other words, you're losing money by gambling in order to ignore the work you need to do to make money?"

Miles paused and then said, "When you put it that way—" and trailed off.

I explained to Miles that he's an example of what I call a "dopa-robot," someone who reacts automatically to the dopamine chase. I said that among the reasons we avoid doing uncomfortable things are fear of boredom, lack of immediate gratification from doing the task, being overwhelmed by the chore or the volume of chores or fear of failure. When it comes to online gambling, I told him that the issue isn't avoidance of discomfort but rather the desire for the dopamine hit that gambling gives. Gambling activates the brain's reward system by firing up dopamine, the brain's feel-good hormone.

I told Miles that men—young men in particular—are at a high risk for gambling addiction, with 10 percent of men ages eighteen to thirty having a gambling problem compared to 3 percent of the general population.[3] Miles responded by saying he doesn't have a problem gambling since he controls his losses.

I smiled. "How are you doing at work?" I asked.

"Right," he said.

Miles had not considered the possibility that the problem is not that he's a bad employee but rather is someone who has fallen prey to chasing dopamine on the job as a distraction from the discomfortable parts of the job. His work involves relatively simple tasks that must be completed and could be quickly handled. Instead, he's opting for the dopamine hit rather than running through the discomfort and taking charge of his daily life.

I already know there's a simple solution to his problem, but I need Miles to figure that out.

"How do I fix this?" he asked. "I'm so behind at work I'm not sure I can catch up."

"Let me ask you a question," I say. "What are you doing with your time outside of the office? On nights and weekends?"

"Watching games. Betting. Watching Netflix. Hanging with friends."

He found the answer before I had to say anything else: (1) Stop online gambling, which may mean getting help. If so, don't hesitate to get it. (2) Get the screen out of your face. (3) Make a list of tasks that need completing, giving each one a name and breaking the list into manageable bites so that as you do them, you will feel the reward of an accomplishment—a dopamine hit. (4) Then get to work in the extra hours to catch up.

Once he got caught up, I explained, he could work on building a new habit: Do the worst first.

"That's key," I said, "and it's some of the best advice I can give. For example, first thing in the morning when you're fresh and rested and better able to focus, tackle emails you previously would have ignored. Do the worst first. Then identify other tasks you dislike most and hit them before other tasks. Do the worst first."

Within a few months, Miles enjoyed work again. The adjustment seemed so simple that he later told me he almost felt silly about it. But I reminded Miles that the foundation for getting tough enough to face discomfort and build strength and resilience depends on making minor adjustments that lead to significant rewards. I don't know of any person who doesn't want to avoid discomfort; it's one of the strongest human tendencies. But pushing through that tendency is how we grow—just as we grow through facing whatever we fear as well.

THE IMPORTANCE OF FACING FEAR

One of my biggest fears is the way I come across to others. This may surprise you, coming from a therapist, but it's one of my biggest challenges to overcome. An example of how this works involves some of my early posts on TikTok and Instagram.

Until the first year of COVID-19, I hadn't paid much attention to social media. But then some friends and coworkers encouraged me to share on TikTok mental health insights from my counseling practice, since mental health concerns had become increasingly significant. I didn't know anything about social media, but I gave it a try. I wanted to help others, so why not?

"Overwhelmed," I said on my first video, "is a word I'm hearing a lot right now. Today I want to show you a technique to give you some relief from that. It's called grounding. Pay attention to anything around you right now that's blue. Say the name of that object out loud. Then turn your attention to the sounds around you. What do you hear? A dog barking, maybe the humming of an air conditioner? Fix your mind on those sounds. Doing that for fifteen seconds will give you a little break to hit the reset button in your brain to remind you that everything going on in your head is not all that's real."

I believed deeply in what I said in that video, but I can also report that I looked like an amateur. Nevertheless, the video got five thousand views, enough to entice me to create more and post them on Instagram as well. Before long I had polished my appearance and messaging, and the little idea to give mental health tips on social media during COVID-19 had taken off. Within a few years, I had more than one million followers on TikTok and several hundred thousand on Instagram.

I found myself getting media requests that led me to look back at those early videos. What I saw made me cringe, given how amateurish they looked. My ego told me to delete them. But I also knew those first videos were a fair and accurate representation of me at that time. And what they showed was my growth.

Using an effective technique for tackling discomfort, I asked myself in the third person, "Trey, why do you care what your social media followers think of you?" The question answered itself.

I left the videos up, and always will, which still requires me to push through the discomfort of knowing they are there. But I do so because they reflect who I am and the realities of my journey, while offering plenty to learn from, even if they make me cringe. Addressing discomfort on issues big and small, rather than ignoring them or hoping they go away, is how we grow stronger for the roads we want to travel.

Other tactics for pushing through discomfort, according to the University of Chicago's Kaitlin Woolley and Ayelet Fishbach, include giving yourself *immediate reward* for the effort, such as a favorite treat (for me, it's Sour Patch Kids) and *reappraisal*, which is reframing something positively that you had viewed negatively (for example, "I don't like running" becomes "I like how I feel after running the first half mile").[4]

You've probably heard about the power of positive thinking; it's real when done appropriately. It's not healthy to overlook problems and pretend everything is okay when it's not, but it can help us reframe the discomfort that we nevertheless acknowledge (for example, "Marriage is hard, but I love this person, and I'm excited by our improved communication.").

A good exercise is to ask yourself what you can reappraise, creating change as Miles did. He didn't like the work until he better organized his tasks, finding joy in achievement as he crossed each of them off his list. "Work almost became fun," he said.

What discomfort do you need to reframe? What discomfort do you need to run through to build resilience and strength.

TIPS

- Remember a time when you made it through something hard. Today, feel the pride you felt then. Feel the strength you felt then.
- Visualize what you want—a goal, an outcome, or anything you want to accomplish. Create as clear a picture of it as you can. Step into that scene, imagining yourself in a movie. Use that visualization as your power when the steps required to accomplish your goal get hard.
- Figure out one small first step you could take toward the goal. It should be a little uncomfortable but not intense. Use your vision of what you want as your superpower to take that small first step.

3

FIND YOUR INJURIES

We men have a mission that is vital to our foundational strength and flourishing—identifying and addressing our wounds.

Addressing this mission is among the first and most impactful work I do with clients as a therapist, and while it's easy to resist and be afraid in the beginning, most men find that this work is not that challenging once it's undertaken because we are built for it.

You've heard of trauma. The concept is more widely known today than ever before, but many people have misconceptions about it.

Trauma occurs when we experience emotionally distressing or disturbing events or moments. A parent with an addiction who has emotional outbursts, an experience of sexual abuse, a childhood peer mocking our appearance, a car accident, a third strike with the bases loaded and the game on the line—these and many other experiences are risk factors for developing mental health issues such as anxiety, depression, and posttraumatic stress disorder (PTSD). Trauma can affect our relationships with family members, friends, and coworkers; our levels of anxiety and depression; and the way we feel about ourselves, interrupting almost every aspect of our lives.

When we experience trauma, our brains alter. Studies show that three areas of our brain that regulate our emotions and manage our response to fear—the amygdala, hippocampus, and prefrontal cortex, are impacted when we experience trauma.[1]

The amygdala—an almond-shaped cluster of gray matter responsible for processing emotional responses—can become overstimulated by trauma and early imprinting. When powerful childhood or adolescent experiences leave a deep mark on the brain, they can shape behavior and identity, making it difficult to tell the difference between a threat from the past and a situation in the present.

The hippocampus, which plays a key role in forming new memories and distinguishing between past and present, can become impaired by prolonged exposure to trauma and stress, such as growing up with an alcoholic parent or in a volatile home environment. Research shows that the hippocampus can shrink because of posttraumatic stress disorder. It can also become less active, which makes it harder to move forward. We may stay stuck in the past, unable to imagine a hopeful future.

The prefrontal cortex—the part of the brain responsible for decision-making, impulse control, and reasoning—can also lose functionality due to trauma. When that happens, it becomes harder to self-regulate, plan, and make healthy choices, even when we want to.

To help explain this, I once did one of my crazier TikTok videos, using wet cement and rocks to give a visual of what happens. Looking back, it was silly, but the video went viral because it explained something so many people, young men in particular, are trying to figure out.

Here's how your past can affect your present, I said. When we're young, our brains are like wet cement. Then bad things happen that shouldn't have happened, while good things that should have happened did not.

Our core beliefs form from those things. We take those events (or absences) and develop foundational assumptions that we carry with us. *I'm a loser. I stink. I'm ugly. I'm not loved. I'm worthless.* These assumptions are like rocks thrown into the wet cement, which then harden along with the cement and get sealed in. We might not even know they are there. But the rocks we carry are the cause of many of our difficult issues.

HOW DO WE IDENTIFY TRAUMA?

I learned early on as a therapist that many men aren't comfortable with the word *trauma*. Say *trauma* to a man, and he's quick to say, "Nope, not me. No trauma here, moving on."

The reason is that many of us associate trauma with something major, like someone nearly dying in a car accident or being abandoned by parents at a young age. But not all trauma is something that big. For most of us, trauma starts with a little *t*, not a big *T*, that is, trauma results from events not as dramatic as we typically think of but are nonetheless affecting our lives, behaviors, and identity—who we believe we are.

I'm no different. My household wasn't dark. Nothing happened to me that was worthy of making the news. I was just a kid trying to find my place in the classroom and on the baseball field. But that doesn't mean my brain wasn't impacted by emotionally distressing moments, in the same way my body experiences physical injury.

That's why I help men understand trauma by using a different word.

Injuries.

Injuries are something we men understand.

Searching for our injuries and acknowledging them for how they affect the way we treat ourselves and others is crucial. Without recognition and understanding of hurt, our injuries will drag us down.

When a quarterback who suffers a lower back injury returns to the game, he will take account of the effects of his injury and how they impact his ability to play. What he won't do is ignore the injury and start playing like it never happened.

Now think about yourself in the game you play every day—your life. Chances are you have suffered injuries in this game, and you must discover and identify them. Studies suggest that more than two-thirds of children experience trauma or injury before the age of sixteen.[2] We feel the impact of those injuries until we identify and address them, turning them into experiential assets that guide us rather than bring us down.

There's even a simple test for whether you might carry trauma from your childhood: Picture three situations from your past and think about how you feel.

First, picture a time you got into trouble as a child or youth. Who is there with you, and what are they saying? Are they yelling at you, or are they calmly giving you a hug and reassuring you in some way? Second, think of one of your games or performances growing up. Is anybody in the stands watching you and cheering you on? Is anybody there smiling at you and showing how proud they are of you? Third, think of a time when you were crying or upset. Who is with you at that moment, and how are they treating you? Or is anybody there to comfort you during this time?

If your answers involve remembering someone yelling, threatening you, using physical punishment, not showing up to watch or support you, or not comforting you when you were upset, or if you simply can't remember any adult being there at all, any of these memories may point to childhood wounds that still affect you as an adult. In that case, counseling can help you look back into those moments to better understand them and begin healing.

Such memories may not seem like big moments, but they shape your identity, self-worth, and sense of safety. While they aren't the only way to know if you suffered trauma or injury as a young person, they could indicate whether you had a secure upbringing with abundant support, you determined it wasn't safe to show emotions, or you grew up thinking you had to be perfect to be loved. Maybe it would explain the loneliness and abandonment you still feel and fear as an adult.

For men, and young men especially, this kind of work is

essential because we were taught not to cry (as if that was a sign of toughness). But the truth is that tough men, resilient men, aren't afraid to show emotion. They aren't afraid to look inside and get help when needed. They are willing to do the hard work to become stronger, to optimize their opportunity, their own lives, and the lives of those around them.

Connecting with memories from childhood is where the healing work begins. It's not that we don't or won't experience injuries as adults. We will, and we do. A breakup or divorce. Getting fired. An accident. An illness. Debilitating depression. Financial difficulties. Or perhaps addictions, which may result in all the above and more. Still, studies show that childhood injuries are more likely to cause emotional dysregulation in adults than injuries received as an adult.[3] Therefore, it's likely that much of the trauma we face as men is a direct result of trauma we faced in our youth.

Men try to cope with their injuries in a variety of ways. One method is through substance abuse, even though self-medication typically worsens their situations and symptoms. Other coping mechanisms include disordered eating, over-exercising, gambling, cheating on a girlfriend or spouse, or other risky behaviors that only make things worse.

What we face is hardly anything new. Such injuries and resulting self-doubt have been around since biblical times. Consider the story of Jacob and Esau, in which Jacob struggled with insecurity and self-doubt, primarily caused by his dad, Isaac. As the second-born son, Jacob grew up painfully aware that he was not his father's favorite. Isaac's preference for Esau, Jacob's twin brother, was evident, and years of Isaac's favoritism toward his rugged hunter son, Esau, caused deep injury to Jacob. It took Jacob a long time to heal from those injuries (often called father wounds, although such wounds can come from any parent or a peer).

This isn't just therapist talk. I know firsthand about hidden injuries, because I've had to hunt for and find my own, examining their impact on my life and how I can make them work for me instead of against me.

SCHOOL INJURIES

I grew up in Chattanooga, Tennessee, where my father was the head of a highly respected private school. I spent my first few years in a public school but moved to another school for fourth grade. The teachers and parents knew me from the moment I arrived, and I suspect some of the students had an idea who I was too. I was the only new student; most of the others had been together since kindergarten. They knew almost everything about one another.

All they knew about me was what my father did.

A first day is hard anywhere and anytime, whether it's school or work. A first day is especially hard for a fourth grader who is the new kid with a father everyone knows. On the first day, our first class was in the gym. I remember vividly how big it looked and how it smelled like kids' sweat and rubber from dodgeballs blending with a hint of oil and turpentine from the fresh coat of varnish on the floor.

As soon as I walked in, I wanted to turn around and run back to my old school, where I felt safe. But I couldn't turn around. I had to walk down five or six steps to the gym floor.

I saw my new classmates sitting together in a circle, talking to one another. I wondered if they were talking about me. It felt like I was walking on ice. I was about to take a seat in the circle amid glances and whispers when one of the boys in the class turned around and looked at me.

"Dang," he said to his classmates, "I'm glad I'm not looking into a mirror right now."

Guys and gals laughed out loud. My face turned bright red. I wanted to crawl into a hole. I felt like a vacuum in my chest had opened and pulled all of me inward.

The little boy who had been happy-go-lucky at the public school down the road entered a new life when he approached that circle and was shamed in front of the class. My new classmate's quip caused an injury that I dragged with me into adulthood. And then it was reinforced during my first year of college.

As a freshman, I weighed about 125 pounds, with the frame of the singles-hitting second baseman I'd been in high school. I will never forget a peer looking at me and saying, "You are as skinny as I am." In a different context, that might have been an innocuous statement, but it brought back all the hurt of the fourth-grade comment, and I remember thinking, *This is never going to happen again.*

Never.

I started hitting the gym. *I'll show all of you*, I thought, *with the biceps to prove it.* But this kind of thinking can go too far, and it did for me. I was in the gym before class; I was in the gym after class. And the entire time I was looking in the mirror at my growing muscles and hoping that the guy who told me I was skinny was looking too.

Finally, it dawned on me that what was driving me wasn't good. I realized I had to shift my focus away from the injury I was carrying toward something better—making and keeping myself healthy. Today I work out for stress relief, goal setting, and maintaining a healthy and fit appearance. But I no longer do it in response to my injury.

Until I did the work in my late twenties and looked carefully inside, I didn't really know that these injuries affected me. All I knew was that as a fourth-grade boy and a freshman in college, those experiences had felt awful. But the lesson I learned was that I might get rejected if I was the new person or if I stood out in a group, so I needed to lay low and stay quiet. My injury taught me that who I was might not fit expectations, so I needed to figure out what I had to change to fit in.

Once I identified the injury, I saw how my assumptions and fears often paralyzed me and cost me opportunities, professionally and personally. I have a voice and like to speak and share and lead. I have a presence that is as worthy as anyone around the circle or in the class. But until I identified my injury, I was hobbled and held back from being my full self.

I'm hardly alone in my experience. Children can be cruel in dealing with fear and discomfort, but we don't think about that when we are the recipients. Sometimes we experience shame and move past it, but other times it becomes a rock in our wet cement that hardens. We don't know why certain moments affect us or why some have a greater impact than others. It's a mystery among researchers, except it's clear that the imprint and damage occur at a subconscious level, which means the recipient has no control over whether or when it happens.

That's why we must do the work to investigate and embark on a search for our injuries. If we look, eventually we will find them, and the healing work of chiseling the rocks out of the cement can begin.

We can carry out simple things to begin the process of changing the narratives we tell ourselves:

1. Identify your source of truth about yourself. That's what really matters, and from this truth you can replace the negative messages that have been imprinted by the injury. For example, when you doubt yourself, ask, *Whose voice do I hear in my head? A parent, teacher, or coach, or is it my own? When I feel ashamed, what am I believing about myself in this moment that makes me feel this way?*
2. Write down the messages you tell yourself and take a careful look at them. You should be able to easily see if they are false in the first place.
3. Think of two things you *like* about yourself—which may be tougher than you think because too often we think of all the things we don't like about ourselves. Then think of two things you'd like to believe about yourself. If one or both of those are tough to believe, they are very likely indications of trauma.
4. Think about the highs and lows of the first ten years of your life, when that cement was still wet, and remember times of innocence, joy, wonder, confidence, and exploration. Imagine bringing those qualities to today and tomorrow. They are still within you and are waiting for you to set them free once again, so you can flourish as the person you were meant to be.

Remember, we can only rise as far as the healing of our wounds can take us. We can only hold down our pain for so long before it surfaces. We communicate only as well as our self-awareness allows. And we can only love others to the heights we've been loved—the heights of the love we know.

We can't escape our unhealed injuries without addressing them. Saying we are fine won't get it done. That strategy has been carried out time and time again, and it's a loser every time, knocking good and talented men out of the game. Injuries will continue to influence our behavior until we find the courage to deal with them.

JOY IS LESS ABOUT WHAT WE'VE BEEN THROUGH AND MORE ABOUT WHAT WE DO ABOUT IT

Take Chris, for example. In his twenties, Chris was one of his company's top-performing sales leaders. He wanted to become a CEO by age forty and had the personality to pull it off. His smile lights up a room, and he is a captivating storyteller. He is also highly observant, often able to recognize someone's mood before they do and to notice subtle changes—like a new hairstyle—that others overlook.

At our first meeting, Chris told me he was a people pleaser and highly perceptive. I began to suspect he had gone through some sort of childhood injury. Though it's not always the case for someone with these qualities, frequently it is.

Here are three trauma or injury responses that may surprise you:

- overanalyzing people's emotions and actions
- tending to shut down when being criticized or yelled at
- trying hard to get people to like you, because deep down you don't think you are worth liking

People who suffered childhood injuries are often highly observant, like Chris. Perhaps they grew up in chaotic or dangerous households. They learned to anticipate a parent's mood by the way they pulled into the driveway or by the sound of footsteps coming down the hall. They learned to pick up little patterns and cues so they could see trauma coming and try to avoid it or brace themselves for it.

I didn't jump right in on this with Chris because, as with Wes, he needed to take the wheel. It was his journey, and I was just there to help with the healing.

Chris told me he came to see me because he was struggling at work, even though, to all appearances, he was thriving as a sales leader. He said he often feels bad about himself and doubts he's good enough to lead. I asked Chris about the people he worked with, and our conversation moved smoothly until he began to talk about his boss, a middle-aged man close to his father's age. Chris stiffened and said his boss speaks to him harshly, giving feedback that feels severe and unfair, making him unsure and unsteady and causing him to doubt himself.

Chris said he thrives on the job for several weeks at a time, exceeding sales expectations and gaining the confidence he needs to prove his worth to the company as a future leader. But then he has a meeting with his boss, who admonishes him, saying things like, "You're not selling deep enough into the company's product offerings," or "You're spending too much time showing off your personality when you could be spending time seeing more clients and getting more sales." Chris told me that deep down, he knows his boss is right, but when he hears the criticism, it makes him feel anxious, depressed, and less interested in his work. Instead of rising to the occasion, he sinks for the next week, making fewer sales and feeling bad about himself, until he bounces back. And soon the cycle repeats.

The first time I asked Chris about his father and his childhood, his body tensed up.

"This is about my boss," he said with a frown.

I smiled and then explained injuries and how our dysregulation usually results from childhood trauma. Several meetings later, Chris was talking about his father, now a decade sober after battling alcoholism in Chris's childhood, divorcing Chris's mother when Chris was in the ninth grade. Chris and his father have a solid relationship today, but he said his father is a lot like a difficult coach who is always telling him how he can do better, sending the message that whatever Chris does isn't good enough.

Years earlier, when Chris's father drank and became angry, the criticism was delivered more harshly with yelling and shaming, sending Chris to his room, where he cried muffled tears into his pillow as his father poured another drink.

"I get it," Chris said, before I needed to deliver the punch line. "My boss feels like my father. He triggers my injury response."

I smiled.

"You've done the hardest part of this, which is looking for

the injury. Now you get to do the work to make your woundedness work for you."

I told Chris that pleasing people isn't a bad thing. Being a kind, encouraging, and helpful person is good; other people respond positively to these qualities. But we can't let that impulse become something that makes people question our neediness or motives or that puts our own needs and boundaries in jeopardy. So it is with being highly observant. If harnessed, such awareness intuition is a benefit or even a superpower we can carry with us after the injury has healed.

Finding our injuries, as Chris did, is a powerful first step—like lifting weights in the summer before the start of fall football practice. We've got to be strong enough to learn and play the game. Once we're strong enough to look back on the past and face the truth of what we find, we'll better understand the injuries our inner child received.

It's helpful to visualize yourself at that age and even speak to yourself, tapping into emotions you felt then. It's important to allow yourself to feel the impact of what and how you were feeling back then. Doing so can and likely will bring up difficult emotions if you experienced adverse childhood experiences (ACE), and if that's the case, I recommend you work with a therapist to help with this process, identifying key events and people in your life and drawing lines between those in your childhood and your life now.

Once you've identified your injuries, managing them isn't so hard. Studies show that practices like forgiveness, gratitude, and spirituality help us shrink those rocks embedded in the cement.[4] These practices tap into different dimensions of our emotions and psyche, calming our trauma response and even rewiring our neural pathways, helping us heal from injuries.

It's a simple but powerful formula: Prayer plus forgiveness equal mental well-being.

Without it, we may struggle, since living with shame and anger can equal poor health. That's why spiritual participation through such means as being part of a faith community, spending time in prayer, and becoming involved in a small group are so important.

After revisiting his childhood—and the difficult years with his father—Chris began to see how those early wounds still affected him. He recognized that his emotional response to his boss was about more than just about the present moment; it was deeply tied to his past injury.

I encouraged him to try prayer. He admitted it felt awkward at first, as it does for many, but he gradually began asking for the strength to forgive his father. In time, something shifted. Chris started to process his past with more clarity, finding space for forgiveness and letting go of the weight he had carried for years.

As a result, he became better at receiving feedback—less reactive and more thoughtful. He could see that his boss's criticisms weren't personal attacks, but rather useful insights. And in addressing them, Chris realized he was getting closer to his own goal—becoming a CEO.

Odds are good that you, like me and Chris, also have injuries. Childhood trauma is common. The US Centers for Disease Control says nearly 65 percent of adults have experienced at least one ACE before the age of eighteen. The most common ACEs among high school students, according to research, are "emotional abuse, physical abuse, and living in a household affected by poor mental health or substance abuse."[5]

Finding those injuries and acknowledging them and seeking the healthy path to treat and deal with those wounds will become a vital part of your tough enough journey, opening the door for growth and healing to come.

TIPS

→ Think about your childhood and ask yourself:

- *Does it make me feel sad or lonely when I remember my growing-up years?*
- *Do I have a history of unhealthy relationships with food, substances like alcohol and marijuana, people, or all of the above and more?*
- *How does it feel to be rejected?*
- *What are my behavior patterns?*
- *Do I feel different than others and misunderstood by others?*
- *What in my life isn't going as I want it to? Who might be holding me back?*

4

DRAFT YOUR TEAM

YOU ARE THE AVERAGE OF THE FIVE
PEOPLE YOU SPEND THE MOST TIME WITH.

JIM ROHN, ENTREPRENEUR AND MOTIVATIONAL SPEAKER

You've probably heard this saying: You become like the people you spend the most time with. The idea is expressed in various ways: Show me your friends, and I'll show you your future. A man is known by the company he keeps. The company you keep reflects who you are.

I like the particular take of the late Dr. David McClelland of Harvard University, a researcher and expert in human motivation, who conducted a twenty-five-year study of the factors that make us successful. The study concluded that the people we regularly associate with determine as much as 95 percent of our success or failure in life. These people, Dr. McClelland said, become our "reference group."[1]

There's no shortage of research confirming that the people around us influence our choices. In one study of California high school students, Dr. Bonnie Halpern-Felsher, a professor of adolescent medicine at Stanford University, found that teens whose friends used marijuana were 27 percent more likely to use it themselves.[2]

Research as part of the historical Framingham Heart Study found that subjects were 93 percent more likely to face depression if someone they were directly connected to battled depression, and that the people we spend most of our time with can influence everything from our body mass to whether we take up smoking.[3]

Consider another famous study by the social psychologist Solomon Asch in the 1950s on independence and conformity. That work revealed, through experiments, how a group easily influences an individual's opinions to the point that people will ignore or deny truth they know or believe conforms to the group.[4] Another study of college men evaluated whether pornography-related peer norms influenced what men consider normal attitudes and behaviors toward women. The study found that peer norms for acceptance of pornography that depicted rape was positively associated with negative attitudes toward women.[5]

I share these multiple research examples because one of the most important lessons we can learn in life is that the company we keep has a huge impact on many things:

- mindset
- health
- habits
- happiness
- treatment of women and others
- success

These are more than enough reasons to consider very carefully who's on your team.

Still, you might be surprised how many men tell me that the people they hang around most don't matter in their life. Their reasoning is simple: What someone else does doesn't rub off on me. But it does. The evidence is clear.

The company we keep is crucial to becoming tough enough to thrive. Life is hard enough without the odds being stacked against us. Having the right people on our team helps put the odds in our favor.

This doesn't mean we need to run away from someone who has problems. Of course we don't. But these studies reinforce the truth that we inevitably emulate the company we keep. And this truth applies in the other direction as well. The people surrounding us give us the opportunity to mentor and aid others. We have a 100 percent choice over how we build our team, just as an NFL team gets to evaluate the players it drafts for the team. Not every player is a fit and not every player is available. But we get to oversee which people we place on our team, which is some of the most important work we'll do in our lifetime.

Your team—those you spend most of your time with online and offline—will make you or break you.

THE RIGHT MENTOR CAN CHANGE YOUR LIFE

My father, Randy, was abandoned by his father when he was only five years old. My father was the youngest of three children, including two older sisters, which meant he mostly raised himself while his mother worked two jobs to keep the household intact, paying the rent and the utility bills and putting food on the table.

My father grew up in Jacksonville, Florida, and went to a high school that faced the beach. He was not unlike other men who suffered significant injury as a result of abandonment by a parent, a father in particular. School was not his thing. He sat in the classroom, staring out the window at the Atlantic Ocean and daydreaming about surfing. Many days, he did just that—skipping school and riding the waves. He missed so many days and had such a low grade point average that he barely graduated.

About this time, a couple of men in the community took interest in my father. They were successful and caring people who were involved in their church and community, and I guess they figured my father had potential but no model to follow, since he was without a father. They wanted to model manhood with integrity and reliability. My father went to college, which was a long shot. He played baseball and football and graduated, and then he was drafted for service in the Vietnam War. He owned an old Porsche, which he sold before going off to war, figuring he wouldn't come back, given that the United States had lost tens of thousands in the war before his entrance into the military.

My father went to Vietnam and came back a different man. Less than two weeks after returning home from the war, he was teaching school in the Jacksonville area. Undoubtedly struggling with PTSD, he now found himself standing in the front of classrooms of students who didn't know much about Vietnam, learning to teach and lead while battling everything he had taken on and left behind as a result of the war.

My father explained to me that without the presence in his life of the two men who began to mentor him before college and continued the relationship after he returned from Vietnam, he likely would have never made it through those tough times, or certainly would not have met his calling. But because those two men took an interest in him, my father had the right people on his team, which helped him become an educator for many years at several highly respected independent schools in the Southeast. Throughout his tenure as an educator and until his death, my father was known as a mentor himself—to students, teachers, and staff—which made him a key member of my team until his death. All this he learned from those men and then passed down to me and others.

I should tell you that I heard this story multiple times as a young man and took for granted that one day I'd be able to ask my father who those men were and then meet their families to express my gratitude. I lost that opportunity with my father's death. With important people in our lives, it's never too soon to ask the questions we want to ask and thank those who have had a positive impact on our lives.

If nobody had stepped forward to help my father, and if he hadn't recognized the importance of drafting them as members of his team, my life—and the lives of many others as well—wouldn't look the same today. It's a big reason why I chose to do the work I do.

I know I can't do it alone.

I can't. You can't. So why try?

WHO'S ON YOUR BUS?

In business, the concept of getting the right people on your team is notably discussed in a couple of enduring books, *Good to Great* by Jim Collins and *The Energy Bus* by Jon Gordon, mentioned earlier.

Collins writes that building a great company doesn't start with the *what* you will do but with the *who.* "First who, then what," Collins says.

Collins's research of successful companies reveals that success starts first with getting the right people on the bus. "The executives who ignited transformations from good to great did not first figure out where to drive the bus and then get people to take it there," Collins writes. "No, they first got the right people on the bus (and the wrong people off the bus) and then figured out where to drive it."[6]

Jon Gordon makes a similar case in his book, writing about how having a positive attitude, inviting the right people on your bus, and sharing about your vision for the road ahead will help take you to where you want to go, to where you are called to go.

"Never turn your back on something that will change your life forever," Gordon writes.[7]

Want to be a community leader, or CEO? Surround yourself with the right people.

Want to lead your family? Surround yourself now with the right people.

Want to thrive and flourish in life? Surround yourself with the right people.

Never turn your back on something that will change your life forever. That's why it's important to assess the makeup of the team around you.

WHO DO YOU NEED ON YOUR TEAM?

Be strategic and smart in drafting your team, seeking these qualities:

- people who share your values
- people who have your best interests in mind
- people who challenge you and tell you what you need to hear
- people who celebrate life and success with you
- people who are older
- people who are younger
- people who inspire you

Finally, remember that quality matters more than quantity. The most effective way to combat loneliness and isolation isn't through more frequent interactions, but rather through more meaningful ones. Many people find joy in solitude and can spend 75 percent of their time alone without feeling isolated. The quality of connections plays a more crucial role in well-being than the number of connections.

It's also important to remember that not everyone you align with needs to be a cheerleader. Keith McFarland, author of the bestselling business book *The Breakthrough Company*, calls this role of the challenger on our team an "insultant."[8]

We don't always like to hear a contrarian view. But just as we need to work through discomfort, so too we need to hear uncomfortable truths. And when necessary, we need to be able to speak them as well. A true friend is willing to stand strong in the role of the insultant. I once gave a friend permission to call me out in any area, and he did so for dating a girl for the wrong reasons. My first urge was to get defensive and rationalize my behavior, but my friend had done exactly what I asked him to do.

Recognizing this, I paused and pondered. *He's right*, I realized.

I have recruited insultant views on my social media videos, classroom teaching, friendships, writings, and more, and while I don't always love the feedback initially, I find, since it is delivered by people I trust, that it's always right at some level and always worth considering. This practice has made a significant difference in my growth personally and professionally. So trust me when I tell you that one of the most important roles on the team you draft will be that of the insultant.

Having someone you trust, who sees things differently than you do, reminds me of Chick-fil-A's goal to address the drive-throughs at some of their locations. Since drive-through services result in a majority of a location's sales, the company has been keen to improve its delivery time and customer service. It has experimented with drone analysis to give team members the insight into traffic during peak congestion that they'd otherwise not see.

Just as Chick-fil-A's drones fill an important role, we need people on our team who take on the role of telling us what we can't see.

SEEKING TO LEARN WITH OTHERS

Keeping our eyes open for who is on our team involves more than the obvious—friends and mentors. Throughout your life, you'll also encounter opportunities to join micro teams that can spur moments of growth and open doors for gaining enduring team members.

I'm reminded of this when I think back to the time I became a ninth-grade high school English teacher. I assumed it might be helpful to the students if I gave them writing assignments about themselves—specifically about the life skills they might be able to learn in my class. For an entire school year, I had two dozen boys in my care, and I wanted to teach them about becoming a man.

They learned things like how to talk to people they don't know—learning to have a set of topics in their back pocket to use for conversation and discovering the kinds of questions that work for almost anyone. They learned about building confidence. We watched videos of athletes in post-game interviews and coaches, and they'd then determine who was making excuses and blaming others; this allowed them to develop a sense of taking responsibility and showing confidence, even after a loss.

Some of the teaching was more practical. One day, I asked the class how many of them had ever changed a tire. Most of the students had had their driver's license for maybe a year, but not many had changed a tire. So we went out to the parking lot during class and practiced. They learned a skill they might someday have to use, but they also gained confidence in what they could do and then they wrote about it.

The students seemed to have the most fun writing letters to businesses. Expressing oneself effectively is important to everyone so I wanted them to learn about how to write a useful and persuasive letter.

THE BENEFITS OF GOAL CONTAGION

We established early on that we were learning practical steps important for every man, and the students bought into it. The result is that everyone learned together, and therefore they learned and grew individually.

What happened in these classes was goal contagion—when we unconsciously adopt the goals of others. Studies indicate that observing other people working toward their goals will inspire us to act for them.[9] Seeing the way a classmate crafts a winning letter inspires others to do the same. Having your friend train for marathons is likely to encourage you to reach for a lofty goal, like climbing a mountain or beginning a workout regimen.

The greater the focus of those around us, the more significant the impact on us. The more we focus and try, the more we subconsciously and consciously adopt others' goals and respond to their desire to learn and achieve. Therefore it's crucial to put together your team wisely while also considering your goals. As someone once told me, you've come too far to get pulled back by people who haven't moved an inch.

That's why dating and relationship exploration leading to marriage is so important. A spouse is one of our most vital and influential relationships—in the first seat with us on the bus, you might say. Having a spouse who shares your values and goals and is also your most trusted partner and ally can make for a great ride in life.

You get to choose the members of your team. You have control over the company you keep, and therefore you have control over the direction of your life.

Ask yourself, *Who do I need to draft for my team as friends and supporters to get to where I want to be?*

TIPS

- → Look at the people you spend most of your time with and ask, *Do they have my best interests at heart? Do they care about my growth and well-being?*
- → Make a list of values you respect, such as being trustworthy and being respectful to others. Ask yourself, *Do those around me hold these values?*
- → Seek team members who support your goals and who have goals you can support.
- → Be willing to learn and listen to an insultant who has your best interests at heart.

- → Keep your eyes open for mentors you can trust and learn from; be willing to mentor others as well.
- → Work on your interpersonal communication skills, including the ways you present yourself to and acknowledge others.

5

ASK YOURSELF WHY

THE TWO MOST IMPORTANT DAYS OF A MAN'S LIFE ARE THE DAY ON WHICH HE WAS BORN AND THE DAY ON WHICH HE DISCOVERS WHY HE WAS BORN.

ANONYMOUS (OFTEN ATTRIBUTED TO MARK TWAIN)

We all want to make good decisions. And most of us think we're pretty good at decision-making. But many of us, more often than we think, employ overconfidence, impulsiveness, or a dopamine rush into trouble when making our decisions.

There's a reason for that: Testosterone—the hormone that makes us men—makes us more prone to snap judgments and reactive behavior. Studies also show that the prefrontal and frontal cortexes—the parts of the brain responsible for decision-making, impulse control, and problem-solving—develop more slowly in men than in women, often not fully maturing until age twenty-five to thirty. Even then, research shows women typically have more prefrontal cortex mass than men.[1]

Layer on top of that any history of trauma or substance misuse—especially during adolescence—and brain development can be further delayed. The result? A significant number of men end up with impaired problem-solving skills and weakened emotional regulation, making life harder than it has to be.

What Does Impaired Decision-Making Look Like in Real Life?

- You misread risk—so you cheat on your girlfriend.
- You don't process impulses well—so you gamble money you can't afford to lose.
- You struggle to regulate emotions—so you punch a friend for hurting your feelings.
- You fail to consider cause and effect—so you get drunk the night before a big day at work just because someone put a pitcher in front of you.

After the fact, you feel awful. Stupid. You are left scratching your head, picking up the pieces. You are probably making contextual excuses when, in fact, the issue is that your brain isn't providing the processing that is necessary to get you to where you want to go.

It's not the only decision-making challenge we face. Too many of us have become like Miles, described earlier—dopa-robots, mindlessly and endlessly chasing the quick fix of a jolt of dopamine, the neurotransmitter released in our blood through things such as sex, gaming, social media, certain foods, hobbies, and novelty. Dopamine circulates through our brain, as a reward, making us feel happy or euphoric and satisfied.

We're told from an early age to guard our hearts above all else, which is great counsel. But we also need to guard our dopamine because it prompts us to seek highs from activities—such as gambling, pornography, games, drugs, online shopping, or whatever it is for you—that can be destructive.

A study by Dr. George F. Koob and Dr. Michel Le Moal synthesized findings from a wide range of existing studies about dopamine and its pleasure.[2] They found that the more the brain is exposed to intense pleasure, the more it compensates by reducing the availability of reward pathways and increasing stress pathways, leading to a heightened sensitivity to pain and diminished pleasure. It means that prolonged pleasure exposure leads to long-lasting pain and a higher threshold for pleasure.

So whenever we experience pleasure, there can be a price to pay via dopamine afterward—a pain that usually lasts longer and feels worse than the initial pleasure. When we repeatedly indulge in pleasure as a dopa-robot, we become less able to handle pain, and it takes more to make us feel the same amount of pleasure. Conversely, when we occasionally experience pain, pushing through the discomfort primes us to feel more pleasure. Therefore, it's important to assess our decision-making. The point is not to dwell on past mistakes but to learn from them and make better decisions in the future.

A man rarely comes to me for counseling without having suffered a recent specific failure as a result of a decision or an action he took. He got arrested. He is addicted to pornography or online gambling and is in danger of losing a spouse or girlfriend. He got fired. He got aggressive with a friend.

But the real issue is almost never just the arrest, addiction, or lost job. These are just symptoms of something deeper—a root cause that has usually been there for a long time. It may be an old emotional injury, a hidden distraction, or simply a gap in what they haven't learned yet, like how to weigh risks and rewards to make better choices.

That's why one of the most important words in your vocabulary is *why*. It's not just a question; it's a tool. It's how we dig to the root cause and break through the contextual excuses so we can learn about ourselves and others. The open-ended question holds the key to our actions so we can understand how to make better decisions today and tomorrow through learning from our past.

THE BENEFITS OF ASKING WHY

When we ask and answer the question *Why?* we have more confidence and satisfaction along our path, are given insight into the how, and are better able to handle adversity along the way.

We are more likely to be motivated and desire to take the best and most productive path when we understand why. In his book *Start with Why*, Simon Sinek reveals his findings from his study of successful leaders like Steve Jobs and Martin Luther King Jr. that show understanding the why is what drives our action.[3] In other words, if you're moving along in life as a dopa-robot or in the footsteps of trouble-making decision-making, it's important to start asking yourself why.

WHY WHY MATTERS

The why is significant because it is key to a sequence that has enormous impact in our lives: Something happens to us; we decide what the event means (the message); the message then causes us to feel an emotion; and the emotion results in our taking action. (Chop the *e* from *emotion*, and you get *motion*. Your body uses emotion to put you into motion to take action to get your needs met.)

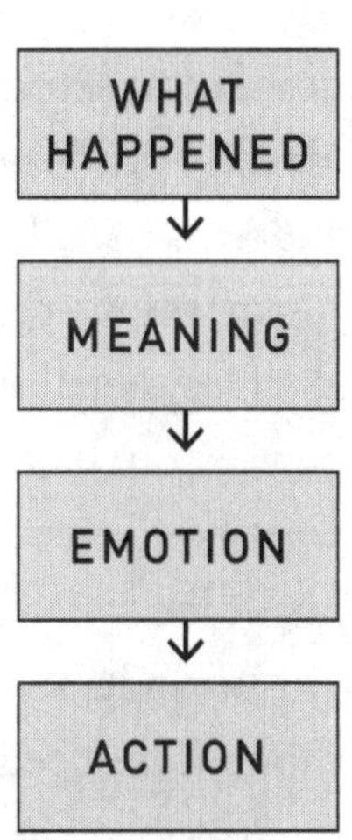

Here's an example from Little League: I strike out at the plate; I assign to that event a meaning—I'm no good; the meaning results in the emotions of anger and pain; out of that anger and pain I throw my bat into the dugout and shout at my teammates.

This sequence can be seen in Justin, a twenty-one-year-old I counseled. He was a kind and caring person with no natural violent tendencies. He was a good student in college and had well-rounded friends. By all appearances, he possessed all the necessary tools for a productive, joyful life. But Justin, a junior in college, came to see me because he had gotten into trouble with local law enforcement. He punched one of his peers so hard that he went flying into a mirror, which shattered on impact. The police were called, and Justin was arrested for assault.

How and why does such a kind and caring young man strike another person?

It turned out that both young men had been hanging out in a group that included Justin's girlfriend. The other guy had said something that set Justin off like a firecracker. It only took one session together to understand that it wasn't the comment that had sparked the violence; it was everything else going on in Justin's life. He had many emotions he hadn't dealt with or processed, and the comment was the final straw. He'd already been worried about his relationship with his girlfriend, who was hesitant to settle down. In addition, Justin's older brother had recently graduated from college, been decorated with awards and praise, and landed in a job everyone raved about. Meanwhile, Justin was making Bs and Cs and unsure of his future.

Despite all this, he had been pushing through, convinced he was tough enough to keep going and make it all work. But what he really required was the toughness to slow down, look inside, and consider what he wanted and needed.

Justin had so many assets—smart, likable, creative. But he thought he needed to be someone he wasn't, which led him into trouble. He gave what he perceived to be a tough response to his peer's comment, but all it did was reveal weakness.

Through counseling, I helped Justin develop true toughness—the self-control to stop, pause, look within, and ask himself, *Why am I bothered?*

Justin soon realized he had been feeling inferior, as less than his brother and not good enough to keep his girlfriend. Immediately after realizing this, he softened—melted, almost—the tough veneer sloughing off. After asking himself why, he gained the crucial perspective needed to assess his strengths, weaknesses, and wants. He realized violence had no place in his life; it was only a poor reaction to feelings he wasn't sure how to process and manage.

These days, I enjoy watching Justin make progress on his journey. He's smiling more, doing some self-exploration, channeling his frustration into an inner toughness rather than into his fists. I helped him recognize his need to cultivate time to regenerate and reflect, to find his path rather than feel anxious about not fulfilling the visions and images cast by others.

With another client in his thirties who came to see me after a binge-drinking episode caused relational problems, I used why questions to help him explore the root cause of the event. Upon arrival, he told me he drank occasionally to "have fun" and "let off steam."

I knew better.

ME: "You got extremely drunk and talked abusively to your girlfriend. Why?"

HIM: "I just wanted to get hammered."

ME: "Why?"

HIM: "I guess I was feeling depressed and wanted to shake it off."

ME: "Why were you feeling depressed."

HIM: "I got rejected at work for a promotion I was hoping to get and so I was feeling stuck and sorry for myself."

ME: "Why didn't you get the promotion?"

HIM: "I don't know, man. My sales were the highest. I guess it's because they think my people skills in the office aren't showing what's needed to become a manager."

ME: "So you're frustrated that you haven't yet rounded out your management skills?"

He looked at me with astonishment, like I had unearthed the Holy Grail.

Deep down, he had known this all along. In his initial view, he'd just been feeling a little down and wanted to blow off some steam. In reality, he was close to having a breakdown. There was nothing fun about any of it. Getting drunk. Getting in an argument. How he felt afterward. He had not paused to ask himself why, so he didn't know the true answer.

Now, it's important to note that this approach of stepping back to ask why can be taken too far, where we overanalyze ourselves and second-guess every decision. That's not what I'm suggesting. Our informed initial responses, when not shooting dangerously from the hip, are often our best approach, giving us an advantage. What I'm talking about here is asking ourselves why about the things we do that don't benefit us.

For those struggling with substance addiction, the why question is particularly useful. Typically, those struggling with substance misuse are among the last to recognize the depth of their problem. The brain doesn't want to face the discomfort that results from seeing the substance go away—the short-term suffering it will experience. So it keeps begging for more, even though the user is suffering negative short-term and long-term consequences.

Take marijuana addiction, for example. Most who use the drug multiple times a day tell me they don't get much benefit, apart from perhaps a minor tingling and the absence of bad feelings. The substance doesn't deliver what it once did, but they still use it daily to avoid the discomfort. They wonder if they are addicted, but they look around and see many friends and acquaintances using the same amount, or more, daily. So they figure, *Nope, no problem here*, and continue to use.

Meanwhile, their bank account is low. Their ambition is low. Their mood is low. All of these are common characteristics of marijuana use disorder. However, they believe their use is normal, based on the people and the culture around them, so their misuse continues without question. Family members and friends may try to talk to them. But this often goes nowhere. It's not until I can get the habitual user to ask themselves specific why questions and give honest answers that they begin to consider changing their behavior. These questions include:

- Why do I continue using the drug that doesn't give the desired effect until I increase quantity or potency?
- Have I tried to quit because of little to no benefit, or do I continue using anyway?

- Why am I not reaching goals I set for myself before I began regular misuse?
- Why am I spending less time with friends and others I used to enjoy being with?

Asking ourselves why isn't just about avoiding trouble or taking steps to overcome addiction. With cognitive reflection—asking ourselves why or similar questions—we receive other significant benefits:

- better decision-making (pausing to consider the risks before jumping)
- increased learning about yourself and what you should or should not do (weighing benefits to your goals and values)
- improved emotion regulation (thinking before hurling your feelings on someone close to you)
- better focus on a path to purpose and passions (saying no to what doesn't align with your mission)

WHAT'S YOUR RATIONALE?

The why question also is a key to a fuller and more contented life. You'll be happier if you can answer why you want to do something.

Early in my teaching career, I coached junior varsity baseball. It seemed like a natural thing to do. I played baseball in high school and probably thought I was better than I was. When I became a teacher, I thought I needed to become a coach.

Then one day during summer break, my dad and I took a walk on the beach. He asked me questions with a listening ear to help me think about my future.

I told Dad I wanted to be a head baseball coach.

"Why?" he asked.

"So I can prove to everyone I can do it," I said.

He responded, "Who are you trying to prove it to?"

His questions made me rethink what had been a fixed assumption. I realized I had not questioned myself about this career path. That moment helped me clarify things that turned out to shape where I am today, professionally and personally. It propelled me on a journey of asking myself more questions, like, *Why am I working in education?* Asking this question led me to recall a moment from my ninth-grade year.

A teacher I admired called me to his desk and asked his version of the why question: "Have you ever thought about what kind of man you want to be?"

I had never heard that kind of question before.

"I want you to write down a list of people you admire and why," he said. "Then I want you to write down goals that will help you become that kind of man." What he said showed me that he believed in me, that he would encourage me on my journey.

I had so many people who influenced me that when I ask myself today why I work in education and counseling, I know it's because I've observed that working in these fields brings fulfillment, makes an impact on others, and contributes to a meaningful life. The why question helped me clarify my purpose, and whenever I feel weary in my work or wonder if I'm still on the right path, I ask myself, *Why am I feeling this way?* so I can get to the root cause of my distraction and refocus on my path.

My work now is more behind the scenes than it would have been had I taken the head coach route, but that route wasn't for me. It was only for my ego, for me to show off to others, which was the only why I had for that path. Asking ourselves why helps check overconfidence, impulses, and addictions and keeps us from thoughtlessly chasing something that won't take us down our best path.

LEVERAGE YOUR WHY

Don't be afraid to bring your why into the workplace. When you do, you become more effective, better aligned, and far more fulfilled in your work. That's more important now than ever. Across all generations, Generation Z has alarmingly high levels of workplace dissatisfaction as measured by disconnection, uncertainty, and pessimism.[4] The men I talk to often describe feeling uncertain about their purpose. They question their work-life balance. They feel unseen and unheard. Many struggle with anxiety and depression.

But purpose can cut through the fog.

Through both self-inquiry and external questioning, we can begin to better understand ourselves—and our work. When we make sense of *why* we do what we do, our energy shifts. We become grounded, focused, and even hopeful.

Consider how companies like Toyota have embedded this very principle into their operational DNA. Their famous "Five Whys" technique is used to identify root causes of problems on the manufacturing floor and to empower employees at every level. The process is simple: When something isn't working, ask why five times to get to the real issue.

Here's how it might look in action:

Problem: The auto assembly line is running slow.
Why? A new worker on the line is falling behind.
Why? Workers aren't properly trained before starting.
Why? Several trainers are out with the flu, and no backup is available.
Why? Staffing was cut after recent layoffs.
Why? Vehicle sales dropped compared to last year.

This process doesn't just belong in manufacturing. Asking why in our own lives and work helps us clarify our mission and avoid burnout. When we work without purpose or without understanding the effect our effort is having, we're far more likely to spiral into frustration, apathy, or depression.

If we don't know *why* we work, we will be unhappy.

If we don't know *why* we're doing a task, we'll approach it with less energy and care.

The how and the what of your work are important, but the why is what gives meaning to the how and what. It's what turns routine into motivation and effort into impact.

Of course, not every task you do will be tied to some world-changing purpose. Sometimes you just need a job. But even then, asking yourself, *Why am I doing this?* and answering honestly—*to pay rent and put food on the table*—gives the work meaning. In that moment, paying bills is your purpose. And that's enough.

Ultimately, the questions we ask ourselves—and those we're willing to ask others—shape how we grow. "Why?" is more than a question. It's a tool. A compass. It gives us the insight we need to develop better habits, cultivate a deeper sense of purpose, and build the strength we were made for.

TIPS

- → Define a specific problem you feel bad about and look for some moments of quiet and alone time—on a walk, doing a workout, or driving in the car without music—and ask yourself why you're feeling bad about it.
- → Don't be afraid to ask yourself questions about your beliefs, morals, and motivations.
- → Ask yourself, *What do I want?*
- → Ask yourself, *Why do I stumble to get there?*
- → Make notes or journal entries so you have your answers right in front of you.

6

THE SECRET OF THE CAVEMAN

IT'S SO EASY A CAVEMAN CAN DO IT.

GEICO CAVEMAN IN ADVERTISING CAMPAIGN

We feel a little bad for the caveman in the ad—disheveled, misunderstood, and framed as the put-upon but lovable guy. He's insulted by the assumption that he lacks intelligence, and we laugh, maybe awkwardly, because part of us relates to being misunderstood.

There's a caveman inside all of us—the part driven by fear, ego, and impulse. And sometimes, that caveman lashes out, hurting others more than we ever intended.

But here's the thing: When we learn to recognize him,

understand him, and manage him, this inner caveman becomes less of a liability and more of a strength. His rawness becomes awareness. His instincts, when guided, become tools.

Instead of apologizing for him, we can learn to work with him.

The caveman inside us I'm referring to is our nervous system, and his energy source is cortisol, the steroid hormone produced by our adrenal glands. Cortisol is the stress hormone that is released when the brain receives or perceives a threat. Sugar is released into our bloodstream, increasing energy and sharpening our focus, slowing down our digestion system to help our body focus while ramping up blood pressure and heart rate so we're ready for action when danger arrives.

See a snake in the closet slithering between your shoes? You are out of there in less than a second—you never moved so fast. See a guy trying to hit on your girlfriend? Snap, and you're there, in his face.

This is what's known as the fight-or-flight response—our caveman response—and it dates back to our ancestors, early men who were hunters and gatherers in a kill-or-be-killed environment. Fight-or-flight kicks in with snakes or at a party. There's no boundary; it just appears whenever a circumstance feels like a threat. The more stress we are exposed to, going back to our childhood, the more active and sometimes exaggerated our fight-or-flight response is.

The man screaming and honking his horn in road rage. The man who shoved a friend to the ground in the pickup basketball game. The man who screamed at the woman he loves. If that man is us, we'll be called a bonehead or a hothead, and we'll feel bad about ourselves.

The truth is, it's more of a physical response than our stupidity arising to the surface. Until we recognize and understand what's happening and make the caveman our friend and asset, we'll battle this cycle, particularly in times of heightened stress.

We all have a caveman living inside us, and he has one job—to keep us alive because, in his mind, we are still hunter-gatherers who are constantly under threat from our prey or other hunter-gatherers. If the caveman sees something he thinks threatens us, he'll sound the alarm in our bodies.

You know what happens then.

Boom.

Are you talking to me?

The caveman is ready to fight.

This is where it helps to remember who is in charge. You are the general, and he is the soldier. He's giving you information, and if you let him, he'll try to take over. But if you ignore him, you may miss some warning signs.

It also helps to give a name to whom and to what is behind the fight-or-flight response that torques you up. You can then better identify, understand, and deal with your emotions.

THE CAVEMAN WANTS YOUR ATTENTION

As we've seen, the caveman's job is to keep us alive, and if he sees a threat, he sounds the alarm.

There are two problems, though. One, the caveman doesn't speak English. His language involves physical sensations. For example, he'll speed up our heart, make our stomach nauseous, or make it tough to breathe. It's uncomfortable, but he wants it that way so we'll pay attention to what he thinks might kill us. Two, the caveman isn't that smart. He thinks many things are dangerous that really aren't—public speaking, an at bat in baseball, a first day on the job.

The caveman tries to prepare our bodies for fight, flight, or freeze to deal with what he thinks is a threat. He is the middleman between us and our subconscious, and he can detect threats before we do. Imagine walking through the woods at night, with limited visibility on a cloudy night. You walk to the rhythm of leaves crunching under your feet, and suddenly in the distance thirty to forty yards away, you hear a rustling in the bushes that's out of the ordinary.

You stop and gasp. *What's that?* Your heart races as the caveman rushes into action.

A bear!

It's probably not a bear, but that's what you think, thanks to the caveman. He is protecting you, just as he would if someone jumped out of nowhere and scared you.

For me it's a cockroach. If I see a cockroach, I want to scream like a child who thinks there's an ax murderer in the house. This reaction of mine makes me angry. I learned in response to go after the cockroach, attacking it with all the caveman's heightened energy, smashing it into pieces while people around me are staring at me and wondering if I'm okay. I'm just playing along with the caveman. He puts me into fight-or-flight mode, pulling blood away from my stomach—that's why we can feel nauseous when under high stress—and sending it to my brain and extremities to prepare me to fight or run, to protect me from danger.

We've all had moments when our caveman stirred us up at the wrong time and in the wrong way. We perceived danger in a school, home, social, or work setting and popped off aggressively to the embarrassment of us and others around us. The caveman pokes us to alert us to physical threats and emotional threats or both. For some, it happens more often or more aggressively, and it's harmful to both them and others.

Sean is a good example of caveman frustration. In his early thirties, he had a solid sales job in medical equipment, was married to his college sweetheart, and had a two-year-old daughter. Sean was built like a Ford Raptor truck, lean and strong, the result of working out four days a week before work. He appeared to have it all and was known for his enthusiastic, let's-conquer-all-that's-in-front-of-us demeanor—except when something made him snap and his anger flared.

"Sh*tty Sean," he said on his first visit to my office, giving me the name his wife and close friends used for him when he flipped, turning him from a nice guy to a loud, scary, and sometimes dangerous man. He had recently snapped aggressively at his wife in a fit of rage over nothing much at all. Their young daughter was in the room. His wife talked about separation and divorce.

So he came to see me.

Sean explained how his wife and friends blamed his occasional rage on his workout habits. They suggested there was too much testosterone flowing as a result of those workouts.

"But I don't think that's it," he explained.

Sean told me how working out helped him alleviate stress. The rage, he said, came from a different place.

It took multiple sessions, because Sean, like most of us, didn't easily open up, but eventually he talked about his past and his father, who was a taskmaster who yelled and frequently beat Sean and his younger brother, wielding a belt or fists, or both, when he got laid off or was stressed about his job.

I asked Sean what it felt like when he knew his father was coming for him. He sat in the chair, straightening and stiffening, his face reddening. I could sense the cortisol coursing through his body, sending him into fight-or-flight at the memories.

I asked Sean about his work, and he talked of feeling stress under the weight of sales goals that kept increasing and the incessant talk of layoffs within the company due to increased competition in the market.

It didn't take long for Sean to see that he wasn't Sh*tty Sean or Stupid Sean. He was Struggling Sean, who had a hyperactive caveman that was inflicting unnecessary hurt on people he cared about and loved.

I talked with Sean about the caveman and helped him understand this was someone he could talk with and reason with. I said, "To get the caveman to quiet down, you must lean in and let the physical sensations do whatever they want to do. Talk to him, if necessary: *I feel you. I understand you.* Tell him you understand the anxiety, but that you belong in this situation you are in—with your wife or your friends. Tell him this is what you want, but thank him for the alert. Then the caveman knows you've heard his warnings, and he can stop trying to get your attention. And logic can drive you in the direction you want to go and help you navigate appropriately."

Sean needed to understand that it was the caveman talking when his emotions swelled in a heated discussion with his wife. He began to practice talking back to the caveman in his mind as a sort of pause that gave him opportunity to think before reacting. "I hear you," he said, refocusing attention on his wife with a calmer, more patient voice and a listening ear.

It reminds me of a line from the philosopher Dallas Willard who once wrote, "Feelings are, with a few exceptions, good servants. But they are disastrous masters."[1] If we allow the caveman rather than logic to be our driver, we become our own worst enemy, particularly when the stress ramps up.

It helped Sean to give a name to the caveman, enabling him to recognize that his system was reacting and fueling a flare-up of anger he did not want. By identifying the source of the problem and having discussions with it, Sean quickly removed violent response from his behavior and moved into beneficial therapy that focused on his childhood and father injuries.

For most of us, the result of our caveman's warning is not as aggressive as what Sean experienced, but we've all been there to some degree. Therefore we can all benefit from identifying what our caveman is up to.

PUT DOWN YOUR FALSE SHIELD OF ARMOR

Most of us men have been taught to man up in times of stress and difficulty, pretending we are fine when we're not. We'll swallow and bury our fear and injuries while the caveman rages within.

Girl dumped you? Man up, bruh, that's life. Dude took your position? Get over it. Move on.

We put on a phony shield of armor, projecting invulnerability, because that's what we've been taught—men don't cry, men don't get scared. But the truth is, we do cry and we do get scared. And we can't win in this life by trying to fight the battle behind a bogus shield of armor.

It all starts with fear. We listen to the caveman because we are afraid. All of us have fears that come from emotions and past injuries. We don't want to look foolish, and we don't want to experience discomfort.

So we distract ourselves or put on a false front to try to hide our emotions and feelings, and we lose the best of what we have to offer. We may look tough on the outside, but there's no real strength to that facade. If instead we conquer fear and discomfort, we become tough enough to better connect with ourselves and others, finding the success and joy we want and deserve. It's not easy to look inside and face up to who we are and what we've botched, and even get real about what we are not. But that's what makes a man, and it's what real toughness requires.

I needed to tap into my toughness when my father died. While I hadn't taken his presence for granted, I wasn't expecting him to go away. The accident happened, and I'm single and suddenly fatherless, and everything changes. It's frightening to lose a pillar you've leaned on and who leaned on you.

I was afraid to shed tears, but I did it anyway. Most days I cried. I knew enough from my education and working with others that real men do cry and don't hold back. But I hurt, and I felt alone and more on edge, with less patience for people, including those I encountered regularly in my life.

I was at risk for the caveman's fear of uncertainty emerging and further disrupting my life.

But I learned during my long, hot summer baseball practices as a teen—back when I dreamed of playing for a big college—that if you want to increase your odds of success, you've got to sweat it out, shagging ground balls and taking cuts in the batting cage even when the temperature is in the nineties. So I had to put down my shield of telling myself and others I was fine. I was not fine.

I leaned into prayer. Studies show that prayer in tough circumstances gives an increased sense of calmness and peace.[2] I prayed and gained strength to spend time reflecting on my father and myself. It helped me grieve the sudden loss and envision myself moving and growing into the future without my dad physically at my side. I discovered that this was one way to keep my caveman in his appropriate place.

MAKE AN ALLY

The caveman can become our friend and teammate, but we must watch him closely. He'll fool us with the emotions he throws up. Anger, for example, is always a secondary emotion, usually resulting from fear of something that is threatening us. To give a simple illustration, if somebody kicks us in the shin, we don't want to show our pain because the caveman has gone immediately into fight mode—and in a fight we can't show vulnerability. So the caveman throws up anger, and we'll find ourselves yelling at someone for kicking us in the shin instead of becoming vulnerable and showing pain.

But there's a more complex way pain can show up, illustrated in an encounter I had with a student at my school. We have a "no hats" policy at school, and I saw a student walk in one day wearing a hat. I asked him nicely, "Would you take your hat off, please?" He didn't. A few minutes later, I said again, "Take your hat off, please." Once again, he didn't. I addressed him a third time: "Take the hat off, please."

This time he responded.

"If you want my hat off, you can come take the d*mn hat off yourself," the student said.

What happened? His caveman had just embarrassed me, the teacher, in front of the class. You can imagine how I wanted to respond. *My* caveman was on high alert. But I reasoned with my caveman, reminding him that I'm an adult and a professional working with young men. I reminded my caveman that *why* somebody does something is more important than *what* they did.

Instead of raging back at the student with my caveman unleashed, I put mine on pause with a couple of deep breaths.

"Let's talk after class," I said, moving on.

After class, the student came to my desk. It was just me and him, and we talked quietly, man to man, cavemen in check. The student told me he had learned earlier that morning that his parents were getting a divorce.

I told him I was sorry for what he and his family were

going through. I gave him a tip on deep breathing when the caveman is prodded, a tip he could carry along with him for the rest of the day. The quickest way to tell those feelings (the caveman) to relax, I explained, is to breathe through the belly so the stomach expands. The temptation in heightened feelings is to breathe through the lungs, to breathe higher up when we are nervous and anxious.

Try it. Breathe in through your nose for four seconds, hold your breath for seven seconds, and then exhale for eight seconds through your mouth.

The deeper we can push our breathing down into our belly when the caveman starts making a fuss, the more quickly we'll put him back into a manageable space. The deeper breathing stimulates the vagus nerve, the information superhighway to the brain that transports messages that help control and influence our mood, heart rate, and digestion. As I mentioned earlier, the caveman's alertness sends cortisol coursing through our bodies to put us into the fight-or-flight mode. But our deep breathing sends a signal to the brain to chill, like an order from a general to a soldier, thereby banishing the caveman to his proper place.

When the student walked into my class, the hat was the only thing he could control. He couldn't stop his parents from getting a divorce. He wanted to yell at *them*. But they weren't available, so the caveman unleashed on *me*. It all comes back to the why we learned about in the last chapter.

The more we understand our caveman, the more we will know about the caveman of others, which can give us more patience, grace, and understanding.

TIPS

→ Here's how to tell your inner caveman to calm down:

- Touch your thumb to your first finger. Now touch your second finger. Now the third, then the fourth.
- Next, do it in backward order.
- Now touch each finger in random order.
- Do it again, and this time speed it up.
- Do it another time, but slower.
- Finally, do it again in random order, and now say out loud the number of the finger you're touching. So "one" for the first finger, and so on.

→ Here's another way to tell the caveman to calm down:

- Place your hand over the middle of your chest, near your heart.
- Leave it there for two minutes.
- This position can activate the same part of your brain as when you get a hug. It'll release endorphins that send "relax" signals to the caveman and boost your mood.

7

CAN'T DO WITHOUT YOU

You have what it takes to help others, to make a positive difference in this world, and to lead with influence and inspiration. And don't let anyone tell you that you don't, especially yourself.

There's a vital role for you in this world with the people around you and beyond, and you have the skills and gifts to play that role. Don't let anyone try to miscast you as anything less.

When we're distracted and struggling, it's easy for ourselves and others to draw the wrong conclusion: *I'm too selfish. He doesn't know how to help himself, much less others.* But that's not the reality. You matter, and your contribution to friends, family, coworkers, and neighbors is vital.

Everything we've discussed so far—the necessity of eliminating distraction, running through discomfort, drafting the right team, finding and learning from your injuries, asking why, and managing the caveman—takes aim at making us strong enough to serve others and ourselves for the simple fact that you are needed.

Most men feel a huge obligation to come through for others. But too many times, we get bogged down in our struggles and think we are not enough. We lack the confidence to contribute. But we can't expect to benefit from our team members if we're not delivering as team members ourselves. Our teammates need us.

WHY IT MATTERS

Studies show that a sense of belonging and contributing helps mitigate mental health issues, including anxiety, depression, and suicidal ideation. Generally speaking, the more socially isolated we are, the more likely we will exercise less, consume more substances like marijuana or alcohol, distract ourselves with social media or gaming, and dwell on negative thoughts, giving reinforcement to feelings that we are not enough, that we have little to nothing to give to others.

But others need us, and we need social connections to survive and thrive. It's the gift that gives and keeps giving, since it's a form of behavioral activation that gets us moving positively rather than dwelling on our negative thoughts and feelings.

When we offer others positive reinforcement and support,

we don't just lift them; we help everyone grow in connection and purpose.

When that fourth-grade classmate stung me, I wanted to disappear—to go home and never come back—but I couldn't. I had to stay. I had to find a way to cope.

Fortunately, a teacher—the one in charge of physical education, activities, and student life—saw my pain. He may not have known the details, but he understood what it meant to be the only new kid in the grade. And without saying much, he made space for me. He gave me a way to belong.

His name was Dr. Robert "Bob" Cutrer, but students called him Doc.

My first day started terribly after my classmate's put-down. I was in a fog, and I didn't know what to do. I felt nervous but had to keep rolling because his comment came at the beginning of gym class. There was another hour left in just that first class alone.

Doc was the first teacher at the school I met—within minutes of getting shamed by the classmate. He came up to me with a sparkle in his eye that showed he cared. He extended his hand, as if to greet me with strength and care but also to teach me how to properly shake a man's hand. He asked me my name and welcomed me. He gave me an encouraging pat on the shoulder, revealing that our time together for the next hour was about more than physical education. I went from being shamed by one person to feeling valued by another in a matter of minutes.

That gym class became my favorite one, because Doc always looked for whatever positive things we did. I couldn't shoot a basketball, but he kept encouraging me and others in the class to do things that don't come automatically. He never said the word *confidence* to us, but he taught it to us, showing us with his body language and genuine connection.

By the time I became a teacher, Doc had moved to the school where I took a job. He became my friend and mentor, an essential team member for many years. Doc's encouragement as a father figure for me never stopped. But having him on my team was not enough. I learned from him that it's just as important, if not more, to be a good team member. I've tried my best to pass on what I learned from him to other students so they could grow in confidence and leadership, no matter what they may have encountered along the way.

STRENGTH IN ALIGNMENT

Hudson Magee was a student in one of the first ninth-grade classes I taught. He and the other students helped the class succeed by buying in, learning to walk into a room confidently, and communicating with people they didn't know. He was a young man you couldn't help but like—quiet, easy to be around, good manners. He played soccer and was active in a church youth group.

Hudson graduated and went to college, following his brother to the University of Mississippi. The next thing I heard about him a couple of years later shocked me. Hudson was found on the brink of death at a fraternity house on campus from an accidental drug overdose. You would never have guessed that Hudson struggled. I didn't know that Hudson's older brother struggled with substance misuse. I didn't know that Hudson's father struggled with alcohol. I didn't know that his parents were considering divorce.

A lot of men try to figure out on their own the tough stuff they face. They think they'll burden other people by telling them what they're dealing with, so they bottle it up inside, leading to an active and unhealed injury. This is important to remember when we get annoyed at a man for being quiet or want to punish him for it. There's a good chance he's carrying something heavier than we can even imagine.

That was true for Hudson, and it likely was something he didn't fully understand. Self-medication became his solution, numbing unwanted feelings with an array of substances, including alcohol, marijuana, and pills. He eventually figured out the substances weren't working and planned to quit.

That day he took the last of his remaining drugs, and they nearly killed him.

Hudson was discovered barely breathing at the fraternity house and rushed to the hospital emergency room, where he was in a coma for two days and not expected to live. The story of Hudson's accidental overdose is told in his father's memoir *Dear William*, about the family's brokenness and their recovery from addiction. Still, it's worth sharing a bit of the rest of the story.

After two days in a coma, Hudson awakened with his former youth minister at his bedside. Len Teague, who had mentored Hudson and his friends in high school, just as Doc Cutrer did for me, told Hudson he'd help him with companionship and support during his recovery. Hudson knew substances weren't the answer, and he was open to getting outpatient treatment to begin the healing process.

Len stayed alongside Hudson throughout. He helped him

find a group of men who shared his values and commitment to healthy living and growth. Hudson moved in with those young men, and what transpired can serve as a model for fellowship and development, for the way men can help and lead one another. In their early twenties, these men prayed together. They loved together. They discovered new hobbies together. Many mornings, Hudson awakened to a supportive note written by Luke, one of his roommates, who used Scripture to let Hudson know he was praying for him and believed in him.

The notes and the support helped Hudson transform his life, becoming the clear-minded and strong man that God made him to be. If it hadn't been for Len, the youth minister, Hudson wouldn't have found a home with kind and considerate friends. If it hadn't been for the caring and supportive friends who prayed for and affirmed him, Hudson may not have turned his life around.

Hudson is more than thirteen years sober now, and he's a role model for many. His older brother, William, died of an accidental drug overdose. But his father is on the road to recovery, and he and Hudson do work helping other young men. It makes a difference, the same way you can make a difference, whether it be large or small. It's a simple formula that works just about every time.

How to Help Others

- make an effort
- see and hear their needs and challenges
- respond when appropriate and most useful

THE VALUE IN STEPPING UP

As boys, we sometimes imagined ourselves as superheroes, saving the world. But it's not always about saving the world in a dramatic manner. More often, it's about the connection, like those young men had with Hudson, surrounding him with helpful and positive support, their faith shining through as a guiding light to help him get to a new and better place.

When a struggling man has at least one other man to walk with him—to help him discover his strength and to offer steady guidance—he's far more likely to make a lasting impact through selfless service to others. When they don't have that type of guidance, they often lose heart, shrink back, and play it safe. The weight can become too heavy, and they try to carry it all alone—like Hudson tried to do until it nearly killed him.

It's the same way with those who are close to you—your parents, siblings, girlfriend or spouse, children and friends. When you offer support by listening and having their best interests at heart, you'll get to watch others benefit. The same applies within your community, from church to the workplace to the community at-large. Social connection, particularly when we reach beyond ourselves to others, is healthy medicine.

Studies like the long-term Harvard Study on Adult Development, which followed a large adult population for eight decades to study their well-being and happiness, verify that we are happier when we help others through our time and resources. Among the Harvard study's core findings are these: Loneliness is deadly, impacting our mental health and our physical health. Relationships and engagement with people are what make us happier and more fulfilled.[1] When we recognize how badly we are needed and how much difference we can make, we fertilize the world and our lives with positivity, helping others while helping ourselves.

It's like the timeless Chinese proverb:

> If you want happiness for an hour—take a nap.
> If you want happiness for a day—go fishing.
> If you want happiness for a month—get married.
> If you want happiness for a year—inherit a fortune.
> If you want happiness for a lifetime—help others.[2]

Ironically, putting others first benefits us. Helping others is about us as much as it is about those we connect with. We're called to do good deeds, and we can't and shouldn't do it alone.

For us men, this starts with recognizing we are needed. We can change lives and community one person at a time by showing up every day like Doc Cutrer did, letting others know that they matter, that they are enough, that they can thrive.

BE REAL, BE YOU

Not everyone is cut out to work with teens and young men like I do, but let's be honest: They need us now more than ever before. Plenty of evidence suggests that men are falling behind—lower graduation rates and inferior performance in high school, earning power slipping in the workforce, and higher rates of suicide overdose than women.

Young men need us to be role models because we can help them find their way. I believe the most powerful expression of masculinity is to mentor a younger man. With a positive role model as a mentor, young men are less likely to use illegal drugs or drop out of school and are more likely to develop a positive image of strength, purpose and identity. It's too much of a burden in today's world for parents alone, with pornography, gaming, online betting, drugs, and distractions of every kind everywhere boys turn. It's too much for church youth groups to handle alone. Young men need other mentors than their parents or caregivers.

They need me, and they need you. But we can't do that just by showing up and standing tall. We've got to be real.

Did you once struggle? Don't be afraid to share.

Did you face fear? Don't be afraid to share.

Remember your injuries and think about your whys. Ask questions, listen, and lead by practical example, such as, "When I get overly anxious, I've found that going to the gym and working out to some inspirational music keeps me from turning to something unhealthy."

Ask what activities they like and engage with them in those. Show interest in their talents and gifts. Perhaps write a letter, like Luke did with Hudson, sharing the reasons you believe in them. Share your own story if it will be relatable for them.

You can change a young man's life, just as someone

changed your life for the better and helped get you this far. In the process, your life can experience positive change once again.

TIPS

- → Remember that you are needed and have gifts that others will benefit from.
- → Keep your eyes open for someone who can use your help.
- → Deliver ample, honest affirmation and encouragement.
- → Keep your listening ears on high alert.
- → Be honest about yourself, including your past struggles and paths to redemption.

8

THAT'S ON ME

I UNDERSTAND THAT I'M NOT PERFECT. I MADE MISTAKES AND I HAD A HAND IN EVERYTHING THAT'S HAPPENED TO ME, GOOD AND BAD.

DWAYNE WADE, FORMER NBA STAR

It's easy to cast blame on something or someone else.

I'd have started that business if he hadn't stolen my idea.

We'd have won the game if our players had come out more focused.

I'd go to the gym more often, but my wife insists I come home after work.

My car wouldn't have hit the garage if my spouse wasn't trying to talk to me when I was backing out.

But the truth is, it's profoundly beneficial to take responsibility when we've had a role in whatever has gone wrong.

That's on me.

We become genuinely mature and achieve personal growth and peace of mind when we stop complaining, condemning, and pointing fingers at others or blaming our circumstances. Instead, we become genuinely mature when we harness our circumstances, own them, and use them to unearth capabilities that can power us forward.

Pointing fingers and casting blame is denial of responsibility, and denial is one of the most common coping strategies for pain. When we deny, we avoid reality. We may achieve a measure of short-term relief, but we'll experience more pain later when reality can't be ignored.

When we show humility and accept responsibility, we gain valuable trust from others and build confidence in ourselves. Others see us as approachable, and easy to work with. They see us as accountable and willing to learn. They see our ability to solve problems and to communicate with integrity and wisdom.

BE ACCOUNTABLE

Making our way through the discomfort of taking responsibility can be incredibly freeing. We feel empowered because we realize that only we can stop ourselves. Even if we didn't cause the problem, we always have control over our reaction and subsequent actions.

That's why taking ownership, even when it's not our fault, is the fastest way to move from a state of paralysis or victimhood to one of agency, action, and, ultimately, success and happiness.

But don't get me wrong. Taking the blame doesn't mean beating yourself up. Of course not. You're a human being, not a human doing. You're not defined by just one bad decision or mistake. Give yourself some grace. It's the only way you'll make a better decision next time.

Also remember that taking responsibility is easier said than done, of course, especially when we're young.

In middle school, I was taught how to do a power clean in weight lifting. I was taught the proper technique, but I had never lifted before, so I wasn't strong. Plus, I still carried all the hurt of my fourth-grade rejections, and I was insecure and lacked confidence. When power cleans didn't come quickly to me, though it appeared natural to others, I started slamming the weight bar down on the ground. Each time it slammed, it bounced around dangerously. After one slam to the ground, it popped sideways.

Crash!

The bar broke a window in the school gym.

Instead of admitting that I had slammed the bar on the floor in frustration and offering to pay for the window repair, I cast blame on the coaches—accusing them of not teaching us the right techniques when in reality the problem was me.

I look back with embarrassment when I remember how bad I felt about myself after not taking responsibility. But painful past events teach us to do better in the future. More than a decade later, in my early years of teaching, I remembered that feeling and resolved to do better.

One of my responsibilities was managing the design and printing of the football program. For big home games, we'd get several thousand fans or more, with former students in town, and the program was a small but essential piece of our storytelling that connected students, faculty, staff, and alums.

One week, the programs delivered, and my stomach flipped. There was a mistake—not significant but big enough that we needed to reprint the programs at a cost of thousands of dollars. The mistake was ours, and the money to print them twice wasn't in the budget. I could tell you how the mistake happened, but it doesn't matter: I oversaw the programs. I had to tell my boss—the head of school, a friend and mentor—that I screwed up.

A large part of me wanted to walk in with excuses: "This person did this and that person did that, and I'm here to try to fix it." The truth is, I was filled with shame because I screwed up and the blame rested with me.

Mentors in my past, like my father and Doc Cutrer, told me that a real man owns his mistakes, despite the embarrassment. When we take responsibility for our faults, others are more likely to forgive and to see us as strong.

I remember sitting at lunch with my boss and feeling compelled to speak up. I said, "Look, I screwed up. Here is the error, and there's no choice. It must be redone. It's gonna cost, and it's on me. I screwed up bad, and I'm willing to pay for it if necessary."

He listened patiently as I squirmed in discomfort and owned up. When I finished, he paused and said, "Well, that's unfortunate. Thank you for telling me and for taking responsibility. Mistakes happen. You don't have to pay for it. Just learn from it, and try to make sure it doesn't happen again."

I had prepared myself for the conversation with my boss with the expectation that he'd react harshly. But he didn't explode and judge me. In fact, he did the opposite. He listened and understood, respecting the fact that I took responsibility.

There's a formal term for assuming the worst: *impact bias*, which is our tendency to overestimate the length and intensity of future emotional circumstances. A lot of men I see in my office have it. They want to quit a job or break up with a significant other, but they're afraid to have the conversation. They'd rather self-implode and get caught cheating or lying to make their boss fire them or their partner break up with them rather than have the hard conversation.

These men are blocked emotionally by impact bias, by assuming that circumstances will grow worse than they probably will. If you want a terrible reaction, then cheat or lie. If you want a good reaction, then take a deep breath. Do you remember belly breathing? Do it, and then speak up like a man and take responsibility. What we assume will be a difficult and awkward conversation may not be when we own up.

Ironically, when we own up, we usually end up with a positive result, getting accolades for our strength, courage, and manliness. Ultimately owning up brings us respect.

TAKE ACTION

Consider the infamous business story about Johnson & Johnson and its most popular and profitable product, Tylenol. The year was 1982, and the company faced a nightmare: Someone had laced several of J&J's bottles of Tylenol with cyanide—an act of terrorism, not a manufacturing mistake—and seven people died.

The crisis didn't start in their factories. It wasn't the company's direct fault. Most CEOs in that moment would have lawyered up, pointed fingers, and waited for law enforcement to handle it. But that's not what James Burke did.

Burke, then CEO of Johnson & Johnson, understood something essential: It didn't matter whether the company was technically responsible. People died after taking a product with their name on it. Trust had been broken. And if trust is gone, so is the brand.

So he made a bold, costly, and courageous decision—a full nationwide recall of 31 million bottles of Tylenol. The cost was immense—hundreds of millions of dollars. But the cost of doing nothing would have been far greater. And Burke didn't stop there. Under his leadership, Johnson & Johnson introduced tamper-resistant packaging, creating a new safety standard across the entire industry. He didn't just save the brand; he redefined what leadership looks like in crisis. He reminded us that leadership isn't about deflection; it's about ownership—even when it's not your fault.[1]

It's a simple but powerful action in times of conflict and ambiguity that all of us can take.

How to Take Responsibility

- Acknowledge your role in the problem.
- Own your actions and apologize (avoid shifting blame to others).
- Take action (make amends if necessary).
- Seek feedback for learning.
- Go forth positively with lessons learned in hand.

TEAM FIRST

I've had the good fortune to work with athletes from major colleges and universities. We hear a lot of talk about the money the athletes make in Name, Image, Likeness (NIL) compensation these days, and it's true. And it *is* a lot compared to times past, when all they could get legally was a scholarship, housing, and book and meal money for devoting their university life to playing for a sports team.

I'll leave it up to you to decide whether or not they make too much money, but when it comes to mental health, I can assure you that no dollar amount can compensate for the mental health challenges they face. Play quarterback for any school in the SEC, for example, and you can expect an unfair outpouring of praise when you win and unfair heat when you lose.

My conversations with my clients always come back to taking responsibility, because it's the only way you can live with yourself and the only way your fans can live with you. Start blaming the coach for play calling or the offensive linemen for not blocking well, and it will come back to bite you hard.

During his senior year at Ole Miss, quarterback Jaxson Dart provided a good example of an athlete who steps up and takes responsibility. While he isn't one of my clients, I couldn't help noting how he handled himself in a difficult situation. The setting was the next to last game of the regular season in the first year of the twelve-team College Football Playoff. Ole Miss came to "The Swamp" in Florida assured of an at-large playoff bid if they won.

Coach Lane Kiffin and staff had a lot of NIL money on the line if they got the Rebels into the playoffs, and Dart was one of the players who stood to profit. As a senior, he had already broken many school records and gained the attention of NFL scouts. But with the Florida game on the line, he did what many fans and media called choking, throwing multiple interceptions into coverage that a first-year player wouldn't have thrown into.

Ole Miss lost 24–17, ending its CFP bid. Dart came into the press room crying. Now, if you watched the game, you'll remember that Florida's defensive front line put enormous pressure on the Ole Miss offensive line. At times, Dart ran for his life. But he was the guy who threw the passes that got picked off three times in the final two minutes of the game, and he knew he was to blame.

"I'm sorry to my teammates," Dart said. "I'm sorry to my coaches. I'm sorry for the fans."[2]

Had Dart come to the press conference casting blame elsewhere, his career at Ole Miss may well have ended that day. He could have cleaned out his locker and prepared for the draft because team morale among fans and players would have been destroyed. Instead, he took responsibility, came back five days later, and led the team over Mississippi State in the season finale and to a win in the Gator Bowl, celebrating with teammates and fans and securing his spot as one of the all-time great Ole Miss quarterbacks, while enhancing his draft stock due to his proven leadership skills.

Sixteen years before that, at the same football stadium, another quarterback gave a shining example of taking personal responsibility after a Florida-Ole Miss game. In 2008, Florida was one of the top-ranked teams in the country, led by quarterback Tim Tebow, who had won the Heisman Trophy the year before. Florida expected to go undefeated that season. They had outscored their first three opponents, including Notre Dame and Tennessee, by a combined score of 112–19. Ole Miss, with two losses already, including one at home to Vanderbilt the previous week, came into the game a decided underdog.

Florida entered the late-September game a three-touchdown favorite, but the Gators offense struggled with turnovers in the second half while the Ole Miss offense was finding a rhythm. The Rebels led 31–30 in the final moments of the game when Tebow led the Gators down the field in a last-ditch effort to avoid the upset. They faced a fourth-and-one on the Ole Miss 32-yard line with under a minute to play and Tebow went for it on one of his patented quarterback keepers.

He didn't get it, and the Gators lost.

The Florida crowd of 90,000 and the national television audience were stunned.

After the game, Tim Tebow took responsibility:

> I just want to say one thing. . . . I'm sorry. Extremely sorry.

> We were hoping for an undefeated season. That was my goal. It's something Florida's never done here. But I promise you one thing: a lot of good will come out of this.
>
> You have never seen any player in the entire country play as hard as I will play the rest of this season, and you'll never see someone push the rest of the team as hard as I will push everybody the rest of this season. You'll never see a team play harder than we will the rest of the season. God bless.[3]

Florida won the rest of its regular season games by almost three hundred points, beat no. 1 Alabama for the SEC championship, and took down Oklahoma in the national title game. Tebow's "promise" speech, in which he took responsibility after the stunning home loss, remains an inspirational video clip for coaches and motivational speakers.

How we handle challenges or adversities has everything to do with where we go from there. Taking responsibility keeps us and our teammates on track and going in the right direction.

STOP PLAYING THE RELATIONAL BLAME GAME

I've mentioned taking responsibility in relationships, but that's just the tip of the iceberg when it comes to those we care about and love, especially a girlfriend or a spouse.

At the root of most strained relationships is blame, and it's often the small, nagging things that build up over time. Little habits—like how the other person keeps the house clean (or doesn't)—can become persistent sources of friction.

- We don't have enough sex because you . . .
- The house is messy because you . . .
- I'd like to have friends over more often, but you . . .
- We don't have enough money because you . . .
- I only scroll social media so much at night because you . . .

Blame erodes trust and connection, becoming a negative vortex that creates more blame and more distrust. Taking ownership and responsibility, however, provides the foundation for healthy relationships.

Many of the issues couples argue about—whether it's sex, chores, finances, or communication—aren't usually about one person or one moment. There's almost always a deeper root. Sure, one partner may carry more responsibility in some areas at times, but placing blame—especially around something like lack of intimacy when there's no major crisis such as an affair—can be deeply damaging.

Take Hughes and his wife, Kristen, as an example. He came to see me because he was upset that his wife didn't want to be intimate often enough. She told him she did, but whenever he tried at bedtime, when she was already half asleep, she said no, claiming she was too tired. They were both in their twenties, working full-time jobs and dealing with the busyness of a two-year-old son.

Hughes said they were only having sex once or twice a month since their son was born because his wife turned him down most nights. I suggested that instead of blaming his wife, he try asking her what she needed.

When he did, she explained that even though he helped by

taking their son to day care and picking him up, by the time she got home, made dinner, bathed the child, and put him to bed, she was exhausted. She said she did want intimacy, but she needed it at a different time, not right before falling asleep.

Hughes asked her what she thought might work, and she said they should make appointments on the weekends during their son's nap times and perhaps meet at home during the lunch hour. Immediately, they found a spark in their intimacy that had been missing. The appointments were a fun way to provide a change of routine.

The change came because Hughes took on the responsibility of asking his wife what she needed—what they needed—instead of blaming her.

As the saying goes, it takes two to tango. Relationships thrive not through blame but through mutual understanding, accountability, and compassion.

You're probably familiar with the phrase "seen and heard"—the importance of someone feeling valued, understood, and acknowledged. In relationships, when we cast blame, we build a wall that divides, but when we see and hear our significant other, we draw them closer to us.

Here are a few examples showing that you see and hear your spouse:

I know we'd both like more sex in the relationship. What do you feel is the root of that problem?

I get anxious when the house is a mess. What can we do to stay ahead of the clutter and get better organized?

I'd like to have friends over more often. What would make you more comfortable with that situation?

To reach our financial goals, we need to do better planning. What are your priorities around the money we have?
It'd be great if we had more connecting time in the evenings. What activities would you like to do together?

Simple, everyday acts of empathy better connect us and address our problems while avoiding blame—the relationship killer. But when we blame our significant other, they are more likely to experience low self-esteem and anxiety or depression, and may even become angry with us. Blaming can be a form of gaslighting, which I'm sure you've heard plenty about. The phrase, while prone to overuse, defines a real phenomenon—casting blame and causing someone to question their sense of reality, their memory, and their perceptions. We see gaslighting at play all too often in romantic relationships as a means of control; it typically involves denial of responsibility and aggressive forms of blaming the significant other. Changing the subject and ignoring the truth when confronted with a lie or some hurtful behavior is another form of gaslighting.

Some Examples of Gaslighting

- "That never happened!" (when you and she both know it did).
- "You're making that up" (when you and she both know she's not).
- "You're too sensitive."

- "If you weren't such an overreactor, I wouldn't have done that."

The unhealthy flip side of blaming and gaslighting is becoming the constant peacekeeper—the one who smooths things over just to keep conflict at bay. It's a form of codependency: You rely so much on the other person that you start taking blame for things that were never yours to bear simply to make the tension disappear.

While keeping the peace by perpetually taking the blame can feel safe in the moment, it can cost you your own well-being—and the relationship too. This strategy buries real problems and cuts off honest communication.

And gaslighting doesn't just affect spouses and girlfriends. It shows up in families too. Bringing blame-free, honest conversations into our relationships with parents and siblings is just as important. A lot of guys in their twenties and thirties think they're totally independent, but old ties linger. Maybe you're resentful that your parents played favorites with your brother or sister. I've heard it so many times: *I've been busting my butt while my younger brother coasts, and my parents keep bailing him out.*

Bitterness builds up when you feel that one sibling always gets rescued. It's easy to stay stuck there, but blame just keeps you spinning. It's far better to open a real conversation. Ask the questions you're afraid to ask. You may not love the answer, but at least you can move forward.

And remember: You oversee you.

Self-sufficiency and taking responsibility will make you freer and happier in the long run.

TIPS

- → The next time someone gives feedback or constructive criticism, say thank you before saying anything else. It'll build the habit of being open to growth and kill the habit of getting defensive.
- → When you apologize or tell someone something that might be uncomfortable, try to imagine what they might be feeling. For example, "I'm sorry for what I did. I can imagine you're probably angry with me right now." It shows the other person that you're trying to understand them. Even if you get it wrong, they'll see that you're trying to connect, and they may well move in your direction.

9

YOUR FATHER (OR FATHER FIGURE) ISN'T PERFECT

ONE OF THE GREATEST TRAGEDIES IN LIFE IS THAT FATHERS AND SONS CAN LOVE EACH OTHER DEEPLY WITHOUT EVER GETTING TO KNOW EACH OTHER.

ANONYMOUS—SOMETIMES ATTRIBUTED TO ALAN WATTS OR MICHAEL JOSEPHSON

Your father is a lot like you.

You may not want to hear this, because, yes, you benefit from having a younger perspective, and you are not him. But the odds are high, especially if you grew up in a household with your biological father, that you have a lot in common.

This is true because of two reasons. The first is *DNA*, the carrier of our genetic composition passed on to us from parents. Our DNA affects everything from eye color and height to the potential for mental health issues, including schizophrenia and other disorders. The second reason is *learned socialization*, which begins at birth and influences how we feel and think about society, norms, and culture.

The effects of socialization are as significant as those from the DNA we inherit, which means that men who didn't grow up with their biological father likely were shaped significantly by a stepfather or whoever filled the father figure role in their life.

Studies show that men who exhibit violent or criminal behavior are more likely to have a father who broke (or breaks) the law.[1] For sons with law-abiding fathers, it's almost a mathematical fact that they won't commit a felony.[2] If your father (or mother) struggled with addiction or substance abuse, odds are higher that you, too, will battle addiction or substance misuse.[3]

The way your father engaged with you has much to do with your overall well-being. Suppose your father was married and actively engaged with you and any siblings—playing ball, taking you shopping, going to a movie, or playing games at home. In that case, you may likely exhibit less aggression or disobedience and fewer mood disorders, including anxiety or depression, than sons who did not have that benefit. If your father treated you affectionately as an infant and into childhood, including frequent kissing and hugging around the age of two, you are more likely to score higher in reading and math testing.[4]

None of these outcomes are guaranteed. I'm only pointing out statistical odds, but what I see in counseling validates these statistics. It's important to have awareness of these factors in order to better understand ourselves and our fathers or father figures.

HAND-ME-DOWN HABITS

Noah came to see me at the age of twenty-seven because he was drinking to the point where he felt like it was getting beyond his control. He had started drinking in high school when his parents allowed him to do so at home if he promised not to drive. He could have friends over, hang out, and drink. Their idea was that he was going to do it anyway in college and therefore drinking at home "safely" might allow him to "learn" to drink responsibly.

Both of his parents were drinkers. He rarely saw his father without a drink after 5:00 p.m. He had grown up in a nurturing family that on paper had it all. He and his two siblings, a younger brother and a little sister, had never lacked anything. His father was a regional bank president, president of the local country club, and a deacon at church. Everybody liked his father, Noah said.

I asked questions about his childhood, trying to see if he could pinpoint any injuries, but the only thing that kept showing up in Noah's responses had to do with his father's drinking. If the family went to a wedding, for example, his father was among the loudest in the crowd, making repeated trips to the bar, telling stories, and slapping backs. At home on ordinary evenings, his father walked into the house shortly after 5:00 p.m. and went straight to the home bar to do a tall pour of whiskey to "unwind." If the family went out to dinner, his father had several drinks. Everything his father did, whether at home after 5:00 p.m., playing golf, or hanging out at the country club on the weekend, involved drinking.

I asked Noah if he ever saw his father drunk.

"A few times," he said. "Not much."

Did he ever see him not drink after 5:00 p.m. and on weekends?

"A few times," Noah said. "Not many."

"How many drinks did your father consume a week?"

"Gee," Noah said, "I mean, if you counted tall pours as what they were actually . . . I mean, my father had thirty to forty drinks a week. Every week—nights and weekends. For sure." (The U.S Department of Agriculture says moderate alcohol drinking for men is two drinks a day or less.[5])

When did you see your father most?

He paused. "When he was home from the office—nights and weekends mostly."

In other words, most of the time Noah spent with his father, his father was distracting himself with five or more drinks a day. On the surface, this experience doesn't sound like a major injury or trauma. There was no abuse. His father was physically present. But heavy drinking distracts us, making us less focused and potentially altering our mood, judgment, and behavior.

I asked Noah about his own drinking pattern. He explained that in college, he frequently binged but didn't reach for a drink habitually after work. Now he's a lawyer working primarily with banks, and in recent years, as the workload and stress increased, he found himself coming home, pouring a vodka drink or a glass of wine, which turned into refills. He admitted the drinking occured most days of the week, and the drinks were adding up.

"There's also the weekend," Noah said. "I play golf at the club, and friends and I usually drink."

I don't have to tell Noah what's going on in his life. My questions are leading to his answers.

"Did your father ever talk to you about alcohol risks and misuse?" I ask.

"Only about being responsible. Not getting arrested. Showing up for work every day."

Noah hasn't missed work. But he isn't twenty-one anymore, with the resilience and stamina of a younger man. Noah says his alcohol use is making him feel foggy too many days, and he doesn't see any benefit from the drinking he's doing. Still, he keeps doing it—but he is sure he's not addicted. Yet he's drinking "more than twenty but fewer than thirty drinks a week," and it's on the rise.

He's becoming his father—less focused on the people and the world outside of the office.

I explain injuries to Noah, and he begins to connect the dots. He rarely saw his father in social engagement without alcohol, and his father was among his most prominent role models. He's likely hurt that his father rarely focused on him but was more concerned about refilling his drink. Now Noah is modeling the same behavior, which if not addressed, will likely get passed on to his children if he becomes a father.

Recognizing the problem was Noah's first step. Taking a deeper look to identify injury was the second step, followed by steps to form new habits, like intentional evening and weekend activities that don't involve alcohol. But something bigger came from Noah's realizations about his father. Throughout his life, Noah had considered his father's alcohol use to be okay, normal, and even fun. But in stepping back to look at his father's life and behavior, he considered for the first time that he was bothered by his father's high alcohol use because it was more about his father than their relationship. And he began to see how he had started mimicking his father's behavior, which in reality was the very thing that had hurt him.

FEAR IN PARENTHOOD

Our parents love us. They want the best for us. But they often parent out of fear, and fear drives both action and inaction. That's why parents sometimes show effusive praise when we've done well, like hitting a home run in high school or landing a new account as an adult, or show disappointment when we stumble, like when we get into trouble in school or lose our job. But none of these events are inherently good or bad; they're just part of growing up and finding our way in the world, just as our fathers had to do.

It's the conversations in between that are so difficult for most fathers and sons—it's the space that can leave us vulnerable.

Take, for example, the fact that Noah's father never talked about alcohol except for encouraging Noah to "learn" how to drink as a senior in high school—a move that turned out to be quite successful, leaving Noah as an adult to unlearn his drinking habit. Once Noah recognized the issue and its impact on him, he talked to his father, who shared for the first time that he'd had problems with alcohol in high school and college, resulting in arrests for driving while intoxicated, and that he was afraid Noah might face the same thing. His teaching Noah how to drink, then, was done out of fear, as was the decision to withhold information about the trouble alcohol had caused in his own life.

This dynamic was like the one experienced by Hudson, the student I mentioned earlier who survived an accidental drug overdose. Hudson's father, David, often speaks to students and parents about his and his sons' experience. He tells that when Hudson and his brother William were caught drinking and using marijuana in high school, they were punished for their behavior rather than counseled for what they faced—inherited traits and behavioral patterns they adopted for self-medication. David was much like Noah's father, a daily drinker in a family where most of the things the family did for fun involved alcohol. David himself struggled with alcohol in his late middle school and early high school years, failing tenth-grade English as a result, but he never shared that fact with his sons.

Instead, when David caught his sons drinking and using marijuana as teens, he yelled at them and ordered them to stop. Out of fear for them and embarrassment for what he himself had faced, he grounded them without talking about his own struggles. He was afraid to show his sons that part of his life, and his sons were afraid to ask their father about his experiences. The result was lack of father-son connection that led to suffering.

After Hudson's brother died of an accidental drug overdose the year following Hudson's near-fatal accident, David and Hudson began to rebuild their relationship with connection and honesty. The result is a father-son relationship characterized by trust, with both now sober and benefiting from each other, which is truly an answer to prayer.

LISTEN AND LEARN

Most of us have a closer relationship to our parents than we might imagine. The Pew Research Center did a study of young adults ages eighteen to thirty-four that looked at the relationships between young adults and their parents, revealing that most young adults (59 percent) say their relationship with their parents is excellent or very good. Most young adults turn to their parents for advice at least sometimes, and a majority of young adults (61 percent) regularly keep in touch with their parents through text messages.[6]

But even when it's good, it's imperfect. Pew's research also suggests that 37 percent of young adults ages eighteen to twenty-four disagree with their parents about their work, and 34 percent disagree with their parents about their social lives.[7] For many, the issues are far more significant, as studies have shown that nearly a third of Americans are estranged from one parent, and the highest percentage of those estrangement are fathers.[8]

That's how it was for my father. I mentioned earlier how his father abandoned the family when my dad was young. His father got a new wife and family and acted like my dad, his two older sisters, and their mother didn't matter. This hurt my father deeply, of course. When my father was ten years old, he wrote a letter to his father telling him about his life. A week later, he received an envelope back from his father that contained the letter my father had written, with all of his grammatical errors circled in red ink.

My father became a daydreamer, staring out the school window at the surf hitting the beaches of Jacksonville, Florida. He graduated with a 1.8 grade point average but landed in the Florida Surfing Hall of Fame and, thanks to the mentors who shepherded him, became a successful headmaster and role model. I respected my father greatly for overcoming the childhood hand he was dealt. But I assumed that his childhood was the only hardship he faced. "Not true," Dad told me, explaining the pressure a headmaster faces at a school that had high expectations for excellence.

My dad could have grown bitter or played the victim from his childhood, but the resilience he built as a boy—his father's abandonment, his service in Vietnam—taught him to carry hardship quietly. He never talked about the war; he just got down to work.

When I became a therapist, I didn't know what he'd think. But by then, we had started having deep conversations that brought us closer. He gave me his blessing, saying, "Trey, I think this is your calling." That blessing meant everything. Our fathers hold that kind of power—something we should remember if we become fathers ourselves.

Two years before his death, I gave my dad a book about fathers and sons. He said it changed him, leading him to look back on what he'd missed and what he'd built. He kept the book on his nightstand, dog-eared and frequently read, until the day he died. I'm grateful we had that close bond in his final years—a reminder of how sacred the father-son connection is and how we can together be strong and open.

THE GREATEST GIFT

One other father-son relationship is crucial, and I've seen its importance in my own life, my counseling practice, and the scientific research. My own experience, confirmed by scholarly study, shows how belief in God and a faith commitment can make us happier and healthier and give us stronger character and self-discipline.

In their study "Belief, Behavior, and Belonging," researchers Brian Grim and Melissa Grim found that "the value of faith-oriented approaches to substance abuse prevention and recovery is indisputable. And, by extension, we also conclude that the decline in religious affiliation in the USA is not only a concern for religious organizations but constitutes *a national health concern*."[9]

Similarly, Pew Research Center data suggests, "People who are active in religious congregations tend to be happier and more civically engaged than either religiously unaffiliated adults or inactive members of religious groups."[10]

I could list extensive evidence from research over the years, showing everything from a reduced risk of some diseases to faster recovery time from illness to how prayer is a lot like cognitive behavioral therapy in helping create deep, positive changes within people.[11]

Despite the evidence, research suggests that only 44 percent of American adults pray at least once a day and that young adults are far less religious than their parents and grandparents.[12] But this trend appears to be changing. Young men are increasingly seeing the light and experiencing the reality of God's presence in their lives. This is especially true of Gen Z. According to a *New York Times* article, "For the first time in modern American history, young men are now more religious than their female peers. They attend services more often and are more likely to identify as religious."[13]

It's because men "are looking for leadership, they're looking for clarity, they're looking for meaning," according to a Texas pastor quoted in the story.

I agree. Men are looking for this, and it's what this journey to become tough enough is about. Often, young men don't know God is in their future. They just know that they've looked around and realized that nearly everything they were told about how to succeed and be a man was wrong. And they're left empty, wanting and needing more. Our culture encourages us to do life alone and in our own power, but I've yet to see this approach work.

We are empty when we are alone, but faith fills the void.

Every man needs to know he is a son. The benefits of being a son of God have given me so much strength and confidence and helped me deal with numerous insecurities and injuries. It gives me something solid to stand on.

One of my favorite Bible verses describes the baptism of Jesus: "A voice came from heaven: 'You are my Son, whom I love; with you I am well pleased'" (Mark 1:11).

But just as the majority of people in successful recovery from substance misuse get there with God, most men I work with eventually figure out that we can't do life alone. The world is too big, too complicated, and too difficult without God. Studies show that actively involved Christian men are happier, more purpose driven, and more involved in their family's lives and in the lives of the neighbors in their communities.[14]

What is your relationship with your father? What is your relationship with God the Father? Is there someone in your life you can talk to who will listen and help guide you in your journey to become tough enough to thrive as a man?

TIPS

- → Ask your father open-ended questions about his childhood, young adulthood, and his career. How did he struggle? How does he still struggle today? What were his happiest times? What are his fears—past and present?
- → Ask your father for his advice on the challenges you face. Share the fears and emotions you have when it comes to decisions you need to make and seek his input and wisdom. If you take his advice, be sure to express your gratitude to him.
- → Expand the role of a father figure in your life beyond your own father. Seek out multiple role models or mentors who

are older and have developed resilience to get through life's challenges. Make a point to connect with a father figure at least once a month, whether you're talking with someone you know well or beginning to explore with someone new.

→ Don't fear faith but be open to exploring with curiosity.

10

STAND UP FOR YOURSELF

You are enough.

You are more than enough. To speak up. To sit at the table. To stand up for yourself. To be a man of free will, character, service, faith, and influence who can contribute to and lead his family and his community.

Standing up for yourself is a learned skill set that every man must cultivate and hone because it's vital for genuine strength. Strong men are not born but forged, and now is the time to work on your craft.

Standing up for yourself means advocating for yourself and expressing your wants, needs, opinions, and boundaries with confidence while respecting the wants, needs, opinions, and boundaries of others.

You have a strong voice. Use it.

The more you stand up for yourself, the stronger you become. Why? Because self-advocacy delivers three powerful benefits:

- happiness or a peaceful feeling
- improved well-being
- better relationships and communication

The opposite of standing up for yourself is being passive and always trying to please people. It's possible that you don't stand up for yourself because you are out of touch with your own needs, are carrying an injury that has lowered your self-esteem, or are responding to societal expectations and pressures.

Maybe you don't think you matter or are enough. Maybe you're afraid of how others will respond if you stand up for yourself or that you'll stand out and face more pressure. Confrontation feels uncomfortable, so you avoid it.

Or perhaps your girlfriend or spouse is succeeding in an area or areas you struggle in—on the job, for example, or on a diet you both are trying. One study shows that many men feel worse about themselves in those situations and battle low self-esteem.[1] When our self-esteem drops, so does our ability to stand up for ourselves. We are more apt to roll over or keep on trying to please people.

Here's what not standing up for yourself looks like:

- You say yes when you want to say no—and you're only saying yes to avoid conflict with or disappointment from others.

- You avoid confrontation and let someone run all over you.
- You go along with others even though you have your own preferences or needs.
- You let others take credit for your work.
- You let people talk over you—like you don't exist, like you don't matter—at home, in meetings, in get-togethers with small groups of people.
- You put the needs of others before your own even though it results in harming your own well-being.
- You downplay your accomplishments because you're worrying more about the confidence and feelings of others.
- You let others make decisions for you; even though you have desires and needs, you sit back and let others make plans for you.
- You apologize when an apology isn't needed; you give an apology because you're not comfortable standing up for yourself.
- You stay in a toxic relationship that isn't good for you or the other person because you don't want to make a difficult decision or confront them with a difficult conversation, opting to keep the peace despite the damage being done.

STOP FAWNING

In his mid-twenties, J. B. came to me as a Zoom client after seeing my Rugged Counseling TikTok video on the topic of fawning. He said his wife is near the top of her class as a third-year medical student and he's a manager at a local auto parts store. He enjoys his work but yields to his wife on almost every major household decision because she's on her way to being the top earner in the family. He tells himself he doesn't have a voice. He explained that he meekly says yes to everything and invariably feels bad about it.

I ask J. B. about his childhood. He tells me his father was a workaholic who moved in and out of jobs, while his mother worked two jobs and made most of the decisions for the family.

"Are you a workaholic?" I ask J. B.

"No," he says.

"Do you enjoy your work as a store manager?"

"Yes," he responds. "Wherever my wife lands to practice medicine, I can transfer and grow with the company. Perhaps I can become a regional manager in a few years."

I repeated to J. B. some of the language I used in the video he had seen as reinforcement for what he learned:

> You won't stand up for yourself because you don't want to rock the boat. It's called the fawn response, and it's rooted in trauma. You start people-pleasing to avoid conflict so you can feel safe from pain, judgment, and rejection.
>
> You have trouble saying no, and you don't want to say what you really think or feel. Unlike fight-or-flight or freeze, your nervous system sees a threat, and its strategy is to fawn, to make you more appealing to that threat by pleasing or appeasing it. This strategy usually results from past trauma. You think you must forget your needs, rights, and boundaries to get acceptance in a relationship.

> Unless you become aware of it in the moment, you'll fawn for most of your life.

"That's me," J. B. explained.

"Until it's not," I said. "You have the power to start working to change that today. Your marriage will be stronger when you learn to stand up for yourself."

I explained to J. B. that standing up for yourself is built on two basic foundations:

- knowing you are worthy and why
- knowing your worth is not built on yielding to or trying to appease or please others

You must first stop and examine to see whether you fit the description.

Signs of low self-esteem in men include self-criticism and negative self-talk, seeking validation from others, difficulty asserting boundaries, fear of rejection or failure, and avoiding confrontation. When we don't stand up for ourselves, we feel anxiety, diminished self-confidence or impostor syndrome, and frustration with others and ourselves.

But here's the thing: People pleasers get run over. Strong men are willing to fight and to put their lives on the line to make a difference. You can be nice to others and support them without letting them run over you. You'll never find peace, well-being and the rewards of being tough enough without learning to stand up for yourself.

Men should not be passive. We weren't built for that. We don't flourish in that.

Trade being passive for taking a stand and acting on your own behalf, because others will benefit from your strength. Stop being a Mr. Nice Guy, swallowing your pride, voice, and self-esteem. Nobody wins in that scenario, especially not you.

In the moment, pause, take a deep breath, and think about the emotions stirring inside so you can gather the poise to speak truth. Speak up, using the word *I* instead of *you* or even *we*. When you do so, you can avoid creating unnecessary conflict and defensiveness. For example, instead of saying, "You are smothering me," try saying, "I need some personal space."

Learning to stand up for yourself is like practicing a sport, or instrument, or working out. You take small steps in the beginning, practicing and learning, adding more weight as you go, and get stronger. Ask yourself what you want and need.

J. B. said he needed a say in household decisions, so his homework was to approach his wife and express that.

He did. She said, "Okay." No fight.

He told her he'd move wherever needed for her residency, but when the decision came for where she'd practice medicine, he wanted a say based on his career options. He said she made a few counterpoints, such as that not all medical practices are equal and that the community has much to do with that. J. B. listened and responded, "Well, not all auto parts stores are the same, either, and the communities have a lot to do with that."

J. B. said his wife laughed and agreed—and for the first time, they were underway with a healthy marriage—because he'd made his stand.

CUT THE CORDS

For a lot of guys in their twenties and thirties, the scenario J. B. faced is one they face with parents. An increasing number of young men are living with parents or dependent on them for some financial support.

In an upcoming chapter, we'll talk more about money, but here we are looking at self-esteem. Humans are happiest when they are self-sufficient. The potential for diminished self-confidence and esteem grows when you need some support from your parents.

Dependence on your parents isn't necessarily a bad thing. The transition from support as a teen to independence as a young adult can take time, depending on your lifestyle. Also, living with your parents for a couple more years can be healthy, especially if there's good communication and role modeling in place. But if the bedroom and money come with strings that make you feel less than enough or bad about yourself, it's time to get out.

Perhaps it's the opposite situation. You are achieving success, and everyone knows it. You have friends, siblings, or even parents who want money from *you*, and you are tired of it. If so, you need to hold strong and set boundaries by establishing limits and terms for the relationship. Remember, the financial struggles of others is not your responsibility. By putting boundaries in place, you can show love and compassion and even give advice or money where needed, with mutually understood expectations. Support your loved ones with open communication and a clear expression of the terms of what you can and cannot do.

If you are the one who is stuck—fawning and unable to stand up for yourself—your perception of others is that they are stronger than you and therefore you yield to them. Stand up for yourself, make a plan, get to work, and get out—get out of the house and out from under the continuing support. You'll feel your greatest pride and happiness when you've earned your way.

It may feel difficult at first, but you can develop resilience, confidence, and independence. You can learn to stand up for yourself and become a man of genuine strength whom others will admire and respect.

YOU ARE NOT AN IMPOSTOR

According to research, some 70 percent of all people experience impostor syndrome—an inability to believe that success or accomplishment is deserved or achieved from efforts or skills.[2] High achievers often struggle with impostor syndrome because they look around and see others' successes more clearly than their own. They can't help but see themselves through the lens of who they were—the young dreamer still looking up at others, forgetting that they've already arrived. But they're not just dreamers anymore; they're doers. The old perspective just makes it easy to feel like they don't belong, even when they do.

When we feel this way, it's easy to shrink back or not stand up for ourselves because insecurity and unworthiness creep in. A little humility is good. It keeps us grounded, but too much of it becomes a problem. We must recognize our value and speak up for ourselves.

Remind yourself that these feelings are normal. Then look back at what you've done. You accomplished it, and you're capable of even more. Find someone you trust in your field and talk about how you feel. Odds are they'll remind you of your worth. If you're fortunate, they'll give you the encouragement you need and maybe a bit of tough but caring feedback as well that can help you keep growing in confidence.

You can also use your skills to mentor someone else and watch them appreciate what you know and what you are willing to share. They'll affirm your knowledge and expertise and acknowledge that you belong. When you mentor, you stand up for yourself and speak up to help someone else, which benefits you in return.

RESPECT FOR OTHERS

With everything we've discussed in this chapter, a danger lies, and I don't want to be misheard here. Men should stand up themselves as they share their values and beliefs—but never in a way that knocks down others. You can speak the truth in a loving way.

You and I don't have to agree about everything. In fact, we *shouldn't* agree on everything. Each of us is unique and is gifted with different perspectives. Your voice matters. But remember it doesn't give you license to disrespect others and cut them down. You may not have liked what someone did to you, and so you had to fight for your own voice and space. So be sure to make space for others. Hear them. Listen to them. Learn from them.

Negative thought patterns and limiting beliefs about ourselves or others can hold us back from reaching our full potential. When we deepen our understanding of others, we also expand our understanding of ourselves. And with that comes greater potential for positive impact.

For me, it begins with continually revisiting my values and asking if my daily actions affirm others. I actively make sure I listen to other people, show empathy for and interest in their feelings, and make them feel seen and heard.

A good practice for affirming someone else's value is to ask yourself, *What have they experienced that is shaping the way they think?* Remember that *why* they feel the way they feel is more important than what they say because they may not be able to articulate what's going on with them. The more you try to understand the reasons behind their opinions, the more empathy you will develop for them.

If your emotions flare up when you encounter someone with different opinions, it's best to pause and take some deep breaths to create space between the trigger and your response. Assess and specifically name your feeling. Is it fear? Is it anxiety? Is it frustration? Then accept the feeling without lashing out. It's normal to feel emotion when we encounter the unfamiliar. But we must learn to manage our feelings without inflicting reactive pain on another person.

Once we can listen to others and truly hear them, we'll stand taller and stronger, and our own beliefs can have a greater impact.

TIPS

- → Ask yourself, *Do I continually praise other people even if I'm not being authentic? Do I say yes to everything even when I really don't want to do it? Do I feel guilty if I can't fulfill others' requests? Do I consistently neglect my personal needs and boundaries?*
- → The next time you find yourself in a situation where you're tempted to avoid conflict and yield to your fawning response, pause for five seconds instead of answering immediately and ask yourself, *What would it look like to stand strong in a loving way in this situation?*
- → If you're frustrated with a close relationship—including those with a girlfriend, spouse, or parents—think about what specifically bothers you. When you talk with the person, try using the word *I* to communicate that you're speaking for yourself.
- → Work at setting boundaries. If you feel overworked and tired, set a schedule for your daily hours and turn down after-work invitations for the time being. If you feel you and your partner aren't on the same page, express needs and expectations clearly. If you feel you're being taken advantage of, establish terms for your relationship and share them clearly.
- → Take a deep breath whenever you feel bothered or threatened by the views and opinions of others. Remember that you grow stronger by listening and learning.

11

EMBRACE THE ANXIETY ASSASSIN

Odds are that you've struggled with anxiety or are struggling with it right now. That's okay. It's normal.

Here's the good news: You can fight back. You can learn to manage anxiety and even turn it into a strength. Helping young men face anxiety is a key part of my work, and it's where I see enormous change happen as they acknowledge the problem and dig in for the solution.

Anxiety is rising among men, especially younger men, in the United States and throughout the world.[1] It's one of the most serious threats to mental health today. Ignoring anxiety isn't an option. Facing it is where our strength begins.

But we can't face it through sheer effort and force of will. I tried that approach as a rookie therapist, and not only was it not helpful for my clients; it didn't do anything for me and my own anxiety. So I started exploring the question of what anxiety is. Is it an enemy? Or does it have some other intent, like the fear instinct of our caveman?

What I discovered is that anxiety, like fear, aims to protect us and warn us about what might happen. Protection certainly has its place, but problems come when anxiety starts to dominate. The movie *Inside Out 2* illustrates this dynamic well, depicting what happens when anxiety takes over the control board in Riley's head and leads to a panic attack. But when anxiety is off to the side, not in full control but mixing with the other emotions, she is helpful, providing a balanced blend of planning and worrying.

Anxiety is convinced it's helping us. It knows it's making us uncomfortable even as we hope it will protect us. Like the caveman's fear, it doesn't speak English; it just rattles our emotions and sensations. If we try to push down our anxiety and ignore it, anxiety will work even harder to make us uncomfortable in order to get our attention. That's why we must address anxiety, acknowledge its presence, and process its reality. We'll never make anxiety go completely away, but that's not the goal. We need to feel a wide range of emotions, including anxiety. It's an instinct we are born with that we can better manage the more we recognize and address it.

I once went to the beach with my three-year-old niece. She saw the ocean as a big monster, with its crashing waves and loud noises. When I walked toward the water for a swim, she started crying and shouting, "No!"

I had three choices as her anxiety flared: (1) I could tell her to shush, essentially telling her to bury her anxiety; (2)

I could ignore her and keep going, acting as if she were a nonperson; or (3) I could go over to comfort her and explain that everything would be all right, that I'm comfortable in the water.

I took option three, holding her close and letting her breathe it out as I explained that the ocean wasn't a monster. I didn't wait until she was completely calm to go into the water because it's not realistic to think we can snuff out anxiety. Author Cheryl Strayed once wrote, "Bravery is acknowledging your fear and doing it anyway."[2] She had to be brave to watch me go into the water. But we addressed the fear as I comforted her and went for a swim, and when I returned, she saw that everything was okay.

Anxiety told my niece that the ocean is an unknown and that she should be uncomfortable. When we think about it like that, anxiety isn't our enemy; it's a part of us. At the same time, we aren't defined by anxiety. We are bigger than it. But we must understand what it is telling us.

Some anxiety is helpful if we allow it to work with us. It becomes a bit of Spidey sense. Yet it can also become a significant issue, causing us to respond with excessive fear and dread or to have physical reactions such as sweating and a pounding heart. These responses are part of what is called anxiety disorder—something more than the natural anxiety we all experience. Here are some signs to look for that suggest the presence of anxiety disorder in men:

- anger and irritability (men tend to bottle up anxiety and then it explodes at work or home)
- difficulty handling uncertainty

- feeling threatened when you're not
- trouble sleeping and having persistent headaches
- difficulty relaxing
- increased alcohol consumption and frequency or the misuse of other drugs in order to self-medicate
- strained relationships
- difficulty concentrating
- social withdrawal—wanting to avoid others you once enjoyed
- unexplained muscle aches and pains

As a counselor working with boys in their teens and men in their twenties to forties, I noticed that anxiety disorder is rising fast among Generation Z and millennials.[3] That's when I decided to specialize in helping men deal with and heal from their anxiety.

It's worth noting that more women, in general, have anxiety than men, but men deal with it differently—often more dangerously. Men are more likely to show anger, self-medicate, or even experience suicidal ideation from anxiety disorder.[4] That's why it's so important to address anxiety early, before it grows harder to manage and more destructive.

The persistent anxiety of men often results from regrets about what they haven't yet accomplished or from dwelling on the past instead of moving forward with resilience. Many feel daily pressure to provide for their families, while being unmarried or divorced can add another layer of stress. Repeated negative behaviors like binge drinking, health worries such as weight gain, or physical changes such as hair loss can all feed anxiety as well. Even the chemical highs and lows of alcohol, the dopamine surge followed by guilt and a crash, can magnify these feelings.

GET HELP WHEN NEEDED

The problem is that many men aren't good at getting help for anxiety disorders. They feel ashamed or are uncomfortable addressing it, even though anxiety disorders are the most prevalent mental health disorder men struggle with.[5] Many resort to masculine stereotypes, insisting that they are fine and trying to power through. But that's not toughness. Toughness requires enough vulnerability to pause, take a look, and get help if needed by addressing the issue and developing tools of recognition and management.

You can't and shouldn't try to power through alone. Research shows that denying the problem through stoicism does not work and that untreated anxiety in men is predictive of additional psychiatric disorders, including depression, bipolar disorder, psychosis, and increased likelihood of suicide.[6] It's a lot to manage when left untreated, but you can do something about it and get immediate results when you stop denying and start taking steps to address the issue and underlying problems.

When James came to see me in his mid-twenties, he admitted up front it was because of his struggle with anxiety. He looked up symptoms online, matched them to his, and made an appointment to see me. Yet James spent the first several sessions trying to convince me and himself that his anxiety stemmed from his role as a middle school teacher and coach with its responsibility for the students and accountability to their parents and school leadership.

James was single and wasn't dating much because he was busy six days a week teaching and coaching soccer. It was obvious he loved his work. He had played soccer in college and coached a school team and club teams for boys and girls.

"I can't imagine myself doing anything else," he said.

James touched his head frequently when talking and had trouble looking me in the eye. He was fit and stood about five foot nine, with a boyish face, blue eyes, a light complexion, and thinning blonde hair—attractive by anyone's standards. But he sprinkled into his stories hints of a different story about himself that started and ended with his thinning hair. I recognized the pattern and asked, "How do you feel about your hair?"

"I mean," he stammered, "I know it shouldn't matter, but . . ."

"I understand," I said, "but you need to say it out loud. It needs to come out of your mouth because until you do, it will continue to come out in unhealthy ways."

"I hate that my hair is falling out."

Now we were getting somewhere.

James felt bad about his thinning hair to the point that it consumed him and caused high anxiety.

"Why is that?" I asked.

He didn't know at first. But as we talked further, it became apparent that because James worked with youth and saw himself continuing to do so, going bald made him feel old—too old for the work. His feelings developed into higher anxiety because he knew his thinning hair shouldn't bother him. He felt vain, as well as selfish and stupid, a hypocrite who wasn't practicing what he preached to students and team members: What's on the inside matters more than what's on the outside.

Still, James's hair was falling out, and his anxiety had become crippling—an obsession that interrupted his sleep, his work, his life. He said he didn't want to try medication that might stimulate hair growth; he felt he was too young to start something he'd have to take for life, and he was wary of potential side effects. That meant the hair thinning would likely continue and that he'd have to shift his perspective. To fight back, he needed to bring in what I call the anxiety assassin—a focused mindset that targets the root cause of anxiety, not just the symptoms.

James had to consider what he could control. His hair was thinning, but I encouraged him to look up the statistics that show that most men will experience some level of hair thinning by the age of thirty-five. Yes, James was affected at the earlier end of the spectrum, but he was still doing the work he loved. His perspective was the problem more than his hair. His hair didn't affect his work or the way others saw him and engaged with him. He needed to focus on the positives while acknowledging the problem.

I encouraged James to write down a list of his attributes—his love of working with young people, his easy smile and winning personality, and his ability to help others learn and grow. Writing down our feelings, strengths, and coping tools can boost our self-esteem and help us better manage and understand our anxiety, reducing its power and sometimes knocking it out.

I explained to James that his anxiety may not go away

completely—not in the beginning anyway. But he needed to see flares of anxiety as a "check engine soon" light in the car. What that light is telling you is that your attention is required. It doesn't mean your engine has broken down and won't work; it probably just needs fluids or a minor adjustment of some kind. The same is true of James and his anxiety. When his anxiety light comes on, he needs an adjustment, a perspective shift. When his anxiety flares, he can return to his journals where he jotted down his feelings and see, *Yes, I'm okay. I'm better than okay.*

The same can be said for you: *You are better than okay.*

This work is as important as anything we've undertaken so far—especially for those who struggle with anxiety. When anxiety takes root, it spreads fast, like an invasive vine in wet summer soil. Before you know it, it has taken over. Everything feels tangled. You're distracted and emotionally overwhelmed, and trying to dissolve it alone can feel impossible.

It's also crucial to recognize that a certain level of anxiety is normal. It's part of the full emotional range we're meant to feel. In fact, contrast is what gives life depth. If we're always trying to numb discomfort, we'll end up stuck, flatlining in every area of life.

I like to use the television analogy. When contrast is turned all the way up, you see rich, vivid colors—bright whites and deep blacks. But turn the contrast all the way down, and everything blends into dull gray. That's what life feels like when you shut off emotions. Dull. Numb. And when a man feels dull and bored for too long, bad decisions can quickly follow.

I remember joking with my Alabama football fan friends

during the team's eleven-year run of six national championships and an average of one loss per season that they didn't enjoy regular season games as much as the rest of us did. They simply expected to win. Overachieving is thrilling, while the fear of losing makes us feel uncomfortable.

IDENTIFY THE SOURCE

I encourage men to get curious about their anxiety and ask two questions when it strikes:

- *Where do I feel this in my body the most?*
- *If that part of my body could talk, what might that sensation say to me?*

Then I walk clients through sets of forty-five seconds when they address their answers to these two questions and let their particular physical sensation do whatever it wants to do. We're not trying to change the sensation; we are not trying to make it go away. We're just observing our feelings to see what happens. Perhaps your chest feels hollow and fluttery. You can acknowledge the discomfort without pretending it's not there. As the client sits with me and we walk through this experience several times, symptoms often reduce. The anxiety realizes, *He's listening to me. I don't have to work so hard to get him to listen.*

The next step, once we have become more comfortable with the feeling, involves letting the symptoms, the sensations, do what they want to do, while listening to what they are trying to say. We are listening for our unmet needs or the needs that our anxiety is afraid won't be met.

Let's go back to James. Like most of us, his anxiety is rooted in fear. He has been wondering, *If I go bald, I'll get rejected, which will confirm that I'm not good enough to work with youth. I won't get the love, acceptance, and connection I need to practice my passion.*

By addressing the sensations and needs in a visual manner by writing it down, James harnessed his fear and throttled back his anxiety. He came to better understand that he works with youth because he's good at it. What's more, he's older than they are, so it's not unusual that he has thinning hair.

His story reminds me of the scene in the movie *Spider-Man: Homecoming* where Peter Parker shares with Tony Stark his anxiety that he's not enough: "This is all I have! I'm nothing without this suit!"

Tony's response speaks to Peter's anxiety: "If you're nothing without this suit, then you shouldn't have it, okay?"[7]

In other words, you are hero enough.

Go be that hero. It's not the suit; it's you.

TIPS

- → When anxiety strikes, try this belly-breathing technique: Place your hand on your stomach and inhale deeply so see your hand rise like a balloon. Do this breathing slowly in and out for sixty seconds as your anxiety deflates.
- → Ask yourself, *What am I afraid of? How is my anxiety trying to get my attention? How can I address it?*

→ Write down the fears and your feelings about the root causes, list strengths you can use to combat them, and generate coping strategies that can help you find relief from anxiety.

12

MONEY WORKS FOR YOU

MONEY IS, IN SOME RESPECTS, LIKE FIRE. IT IS A VERY EXCELLENT SERVANT, BUT A TERRIBLE MASTER.

P. T. BARNUM, AMERICAN SHOWMAN

Money may not be the root of all evil, but for many young men, it's a major source of stress, pressure, and distraction. The problem starts when their goal becomes getting rich as fast as possible, an obsession that often backfires. Instead of building real financial stability, we get pushed further away from it. What's worse, chasing money for its own sake makes it harder to earn, manage, and keep it. The obsession with getting rich fast may well be the very thing that stops us from building true wealth.

In the decade-plus that I've had my counseling practice, I've watched young men become increasingly obsessed with and even panicked about money and possessions, an obsession that begins for many in high school and college. Just about every young man I work with brings a wealth of issues and anxieties about money, and many delay getting the very thing they want by adopting the wrong approach to money.

Many of you know exactly what I'm talking about. One recent study shows that more than 50 percent of men ages forty-four to fifty-nine report money as a stressor.[1] What I hear from clients gets framed in different ways but ends up in the same place:

- *Money is making me crazy.*
- *I'm not getting it fast enough.*
- *Dude got his overnight. Why isn't that happening for me?*
- *Whatever it takes to get it, I'll do it.*
- *It's so easy that I look dumb if I can't figure it out.*
- *You aren't anything if you aren't rich.*

Young men are dealing with these attitudes and a whole lot more. It's crypto, investing apps, and online gambling on the smartphone. It's meme stocks and stories of guys who got rich in minutes or hours. Side hustles. Hustle hustles. Sell drugs. Rip someone off. For many, no guardrails or ethics apply in the face of the obsession with money. They see money as an expectation and a validation of them as a man.

There are multiple reasons for this, chief among them

being social media, replete with promises of getting rich geared to preteen and teen boys, so fast money seems normal, a rite of passage, so to speak. There's also the trend showing that young men face stagnant wages compared to other segments of society. They look at their father or father figure and wonder, *Can I make that kind of money too? I've got to get rich quickly!*

Alternatively, they look at their father or father figure and see how hard they work and think, *Why would I do all that when I can get rich quickly and tons more easily without slaving away for years with life passing me by?*

Inflation hasn't helped. Food costs more. College costs keep going up. Housing costs more. Beginning salaries for young adults aren't paying enough, which means more emotional instability in a high-cost environment. Consider one recent survey that showed only 20 percent of Gen Z and 21 percent of millennials feel secure financially.[2] With two out of every ten young adults feeling insecure with money, the odds increase for irrational thinking. Then we open our phones, and scams prey on that vulnerability and distract us from doing what we need to do to take care of our financial situation and future—the things we need to do to feel secure.

The combination of social media, online access, and get-rich-quick schemes and shifting culture and economics arrived in perfect storm for young men facing increased pressure and issues around money due to stagnant wages, expectations to have it figured out and conquered, and higher costs of living. And many face the additional burden of student debt from loans and credit cards used to get through college.

In short, it's understandable why young men feel this

pressure, but the dangers lurking in obsessing over getting rich quick are many:

- You'll lose whatever money you do earn chasing bad and risky investments.
- You'll find that risk and losses take a mental health toll, shaking confidence and increasing your feelings of insecurity and anxiety.
- You'll waste precious time staring online as you wait for the results.
- You'll have delayed taking the time-tested steps toward financial security and wealth-building.

IF IT LOOKS TOO GOOD TO BE TRUE, IT PROBABLY IS

No shortage of bold promises exists on social media about how to get rich quick. Influencers hype multilevel marketing (MLM) schemes in which someone sells products and recruits other people to be new distributors. Cryptocurrency investing and day trading strategies are sold as fast tracks to wealth. But here's the truth: For most people, these paths don't work. They're high-risk, often misleading, and almost never as easy or profitable as they seem.

This pressure affects a lot of young men. Take Bennett, age twenty-nine, who works as a regional sales manager at a food distribution company and is doing well for his age, earning just over $100,000 a year. He was saving money but hadn't yet achieved his goal of buying a home. Bennett started feeling left behind as friends bought houses, built man caves, and posted about their new toys—jet skis, motorcycles, you name it. So when he saw an influencer bragging about day trading stocks, he decided to give it a shot with the money he'd been saving for a house.

The problem? He wasn't an investing expert. Like many amateur traders, he bought stocks high out of FOMO and sold them low out of fear. He bet big on a risky small company and lost. Its stock went to zero. On top of that, day trading consumed his attention. He was glued to his phone, distracted from the job he had once thrived in.

By the time Bennett came to see me, he had lost not just his savings but also his momentum. His once-promising career was in danger. I helped him look back at what he had been chasing and what he was achieving before he got distracted. He was accruing money and growing professionally, following his instincts until being derailed by pursuing the easy path that rarely pays off.

Remember this: There isn't much good involving money that happens overnight. With time, patience, and a consistent plan, good things with money can take place. When good fortune adds to that, as sometimes occurs, the result is wealth.

To be sure, we've all heard stories of people who made millions overnight as a viral sensation or as an early investor in bitcoin. And sometimes you get lucky without a plan. Sometimes shooting from the hip hits the bull's-eye. But more often than not, anxious, erratic, and pursuing behavior around money only results in more unrest, more unpredictability, and more pursuing that ends up providing us with less, not more.

Making money can be good, but only when we carefully manage our plans and emotions. All investment involves risk, and taking risk with money and in life can be good when thought and strategy are behind it—it's *calculated* risk. We carefully study a situation and consider the risks and rewards. We conclude that the potential benefits outweigh the risks and then we place a bet.

Take crypto, for example. A lot of people became rich because they got in early. Bitcoin and other cryptocurrencies are real and here to stay, and they've been a great investment for many, like good stocks or real estate. But much of the easy money has been made. Bitcoin no longer sells for a dollar. Whether it's a good investment depends on you and your goals. Betting all our savings on a meme coin because social media influencers say it's hot and will make us rich is not a strategy.

When we obsess over something, we take fewer positive actions elsewhere in our lives. And when we chase the easy route to our goals, we increase our risk of getting stuck, or worse, because we miss the steady growth opportunities. Put simply, while we think money will make us, it may well break us instead. And yet a study showed that between 40 and 45 percent of Gen Zers and millennials are "obsessed with the idea of being rich" and suffer from financial dysmorphia, the gap between perceived financial status and actual financial reality.[3]

For example, say you earn $80,000 at age thirty-five, which is above average in the US, but you think you're supposed to have a better lifestyle, with a bigger house, a more expensive car, and more toys, vacations, and investments. You'd need to earn $250,000 to have all those things, so you max out credit cards and make risky decisions to get there. Or you suffer from the opposite.: You earn $175,000 annually yet feel like it's not enough, so you live like a miser and don't enjoy your money.

That's no way to live. As the old saying goes, "Don't work for the money; let the money work for you."

THINGS DON'T MAKE A MAN

When he walked into my office, Cameron, age twenty-four, was wanting more. I'd have thought he was forty-four by the way he was carrying the frustration I'm used to seeing in middle-aged men. He was two years out of college, having earned a degree in finance. And it seemed he had gone on to get a master's degree in anger over the previous twenty-four months.

He made a list of all the things he had accumulated over two years, including a fiancée, a nice house well beyond the average starter home with big TVs in every room, a fully loaded new pickup truck, and a new side-by-side vehicle in the garage for hunting season. "I make six-figures. I do what I want to do, and nobody gets in the way of that, Cameron said. "But what's wrong with me? I don't feel right."

"What do you think it is?"

"I can't stop thinking about the Tom Brady interview on *60 Minutes*," he said. "Brady listed off all his accomplishments, like Super Bowl wins and things, but said it wasn't enough." I looked up Brady's quote from the TV interview and read it to Cameron. "Why do I have three Super Bowl rings and still think there's something greater out there for me?" Brady said. "I mean, maybe a lot of people would say, 'Hey man, this is what is.' I reached my goal, my dream, my life. Me, I think: 'God, it's gotta be more than this.' I mean this can't be what it's all cracked up to be."[4]

"Yeah," Cameron said, "That's it. I remember the look on his face. He looked confused, almost stunned. That's me. I'm with him. There's gotta be more to life." He paused. "I'm bored with these things. I'm empty."

Cameron had chased everything and come up empty. He was, like many of us, raised in a culture that says the two most important values in life are personal peace and prosperity—a life where we aren't bothered and where we have abundant material possessions.

Comfort and material gain are sold like the Holy Grail from which to drink life. And yet they are most assuredly not. When men are hollowed out and unsure about why they get up in the morning, they figure out quickly that pursuing comfort and material possessions is appealing on the surface but hollow underneath.

Some call this endless pursuit "running on the hamster wheel"—relentless work, going around and around chasing nothing. You work your butt off and end up in the same place you started.

It was the same for a wealthy business owner named Chip, age thirty-two. The money had come fast, starting when he was twenty-five. The first time he came to me, he was a little nervous and very polite. We chatted, breaking the ice. After a few minutes, he took out his car keys and slammed them on the table.

"It's a Lamborghini," he said. "In the parking lot."

Chip listed a few other possessions, such as a new

motorcycle. Trips he has taken around the world. A gorgeous girlfriend.

"Why the [bleep] am I still not happy?"

He was just like Cameron—in fact, just like most of the guys I see. Emotionally bankrupt, with a hole that money can't fill and yet it's exactly what they're chasing. We were told that money will make us happy, but it doesn't. The problem is that this idea is so deeply rooted in us it's not easy to let go.

Think about it. We make money and collect things that gain us attention from our parents, girlfriend, or spouse. If we have children, they love things too. Daddy brings home expensive toys, and he gets lots of attention. We learned to chase money and things, and other people learn to chase our money and things. But it's never enough for any of us.

Chip was single, but his financial success set him apart from the other guys in his age group. He was called the most eligible bachelor in his community. It became his identity—an identity he didn't want to let go of. But it didn't give anything in return. If anything, it took away from him because the hamster wheel kept going around and around, and he couldn't get off.

Chip talked about how from middle school on, he had been drawn to the attention he received from winning awards in sports or earning good grades. The financial rewards from business success were the same. See my car, see my trophies—my girlfriend, house, car.

Even though Chip's personal life was in a downward spiral, he couldn't give up his chasing because he didn't have a backup plan. He was scared, unsure of where to turn.

"People would think I'm a fool to walk away from it all at thirty-two," Chip said. "And would what I do anyway?"

"What do you think some other alternatives might be?"

I let him think about the answer until he was ready. It took several more sessions.

"I decided to give church a try," Chip told me.

Bingo.

Chip's job wasn't the problem. Neither was the money he made. The problem was Chip's perspective.

Money, when used wisely, can be a powerful force for good. As we grow into manhood, we come to discover that the goal isn't just to earn money; it's to make money work for us. This shift in mindset is everything because to be truly happy, we need three things:

- growth
- generosity
- gratitude

Money can support both growth and giving, and these aspects are most powerful when rooted in gratitude. When we're thankful for what we have, we start using what we've earned to build a fuller, more meaningful life.

CAN MONEY BUY HAPPINESS?

Tell someone who grew up in poverty that money can't buy happiness, and they may laugh in your face. There's a strong link between poverty and mental health issues, both as a cause and a consequence. Impoverished adults are more likely to suffer from major depression, anxiety, and other psychological distress, including suicide.[5]

Working hard and smart to escape poverty to have the life you want and to help others with your resources is a worthy endeavor. Studies show that money can to some extent bring us peace and satisfaction, reduce anxiety and fear, and deliver feelings of contentment with resources.[6]

With higher income and net worth usually come greater freedom and choices, which are desirable things. But it also demonstrates that money is a means rather than an end. It's not riches we want, but rather the things that wealth allows us to do. But if we get the order backward, we are setting ourselves up for trouble.

Hospice nurse Suzanne O'Brien, who worked for more than twenty years with dying patients, wrote an article for CNBC about the hundreds of deathbed regrets she heard, which all shared similar themes. None of these had anything to do with wishing they would have had more money.

According to O'Brien, the most common regrets shared at deathbeds are these:

- I regret not following my heart and finding my true purpose.
- I regret not having the courage to love others fully.
- I regret not having the courage to let others love me fully.
- I regret that I judged myself so much and didn't love myself more.[7]

Many young people feel invincible and can't relate to deathbed thoughts. But the sentiments O'Brien shared are actually true for people of any age. That's why Cameron, Chip, and nearly everyone I work with battle the same problem. Money's power has long lured us.

The battle is much harder today, thanks to a social media culture that idolizes influencers and feeds us exactly what we want to hear. Algorithms flood our feeds with content that plays to our curiosity—until curiosity turns into obsession, confusion, and distraction. And in the process, you drift further from your values, your peace, and the things that really matter in your life.

Consider online gambling. Ask someone if they want to invest their money badly while being distracted from doing anything productive with their time, and they'd say, " No, no way! That's a bad investment."

But young men do it all the time. They struggle with online gambling—sports gambling in particular—which has been normalized and legalized. I believe it is the most significant addiction problem this generation faces, and it's only beginning. Starting in high school, if not earlier, students are losing money and time they don't have because gambling opportunities are at their fingertips. All while at the family dinner table, young men can easily make deposits and bets on the next first down or the score at the end of the quarter without anyone even knowing. It'll stoke their dopamine, begging them to come back for more in much the same way drugs do.

One study showed 10 percent of men ages eighteen to thirty show signs of problem gambling compared to 3 percent of the general population.[8] Another study shows that young men, ages eighteen to twenty-four, are more likely to "chase" losses in gambling, losing more money they don't have.[9] Just as with substance misuse, it's not that they are bad or stupid; it's that gambling is addictive. The system is set up to make us chase losses.

I worked with Mike, a sophomore in college, who connected with me after his mother figured out he had been stealing from her checking account and selling her gold jewelry at a local pawn shop. In one year, he pilfered nearly ten thousand dollars that wasn't his. His mom thought he had a drug problem, but he explained that he barely drinks at all, that he's one of the "good guys"—failing to recognize that gambling addiction is a behavior similar to substance misuse. Nor did he realize he was addicted to gambling; after all, most of his friends did the same thing.

"I knew I needed to stop," he told me. "I just wanted to make up what I had lost and then quit."

I explained to Mike that addiction is defined by someone returning to behavior that is damaging, despite the consequences.

"How did you feel about stealing from your mother?"

"Awful," he said.

"How many times did you do it?"

"Dozens," he explained. "I'd try to keep it to small amounts so she wouldn't notice. And so I could try to stop there. But I kept coming back for more."

That's addictive behavior.

Casinos and electronic casino games are built and wired for this—to lure our brains into addictive behavior. The house always wins.

CHASING LOSSES NEVER WINS

Gambling zaps us in two big areas of vulnerability: money idolatry and an adrenaline rush. When someone who doesn't have a gambling problem loses money, their brain tells them to stop playing. *Get away!* But for those who have a problem, losing money triggers the urge to play more. It's a phenomenon called "chasing losses." The gambling industry knows how to manipulate us to get us to do it. For example, casinos often purposefully vary the volume, length, and size of the jingling sounds and the flashing lights to increase our excitement and make us overestimate how much we are winning.

Gambling boosts our mood, which makes us feel more excited and optimistic that we can win. And when we don't win, we're purposefully given near misses because research shows that almost winning triggers a more substantial urge to play than even winning itself.[10] We're given just enough wins to make us think we have skills and can beat the odds. And yet the whole time they are making our brain their puppet, so we'll play longer and lay down more money than we planned. We keep losing, and by the end, we're depressed and feel bad about ourselves.

We may win some along the way. We may win big. And that's a problem. One win means we'll chase the win and end up with bigger losses. That's how we get in over our heads into gambling addiction. It's the same with substances. Nobody ever means to get addicted. We mean to control it, and we see others control it. And yet we can't.

There's a similar dynamic with online scams, the promises of getting-rich quick schemes that entice you to send them your money. Gen Zers are more than twice as likely as boomers to fall victim to an online scam, according to a Deloitte report.[11] Spend more than four hours a day on social media and odds increase that you'll get exposed to scams promising too-good-to-be-true returns on money and fall for one.

The good news is that there is help for gambling addiction just as with substance addiction, through counselors and treatments centers, depending on what you need. There's also help for online addiction. You can fight back and win. Don't let them make your brain their puppet. With help, you can flip the odds in your favor. But you can't delay.

People under forty grew up in what Jennifer Breheny Wallace calls in her book *Never Enough* "professionalized childhood," with our value based on how much we achieved in grades, athletic feats, and scholarships won.[12] We distract ourselves online, where we are shown "perfect" bodies and fed get-rich-quick schemes that pull us further down. When it comes to money, and to our lives, we must take charge.

Our happiness and financial success are in our hands.

TIME-TESTED WEALTH BUILDING

What we're not told online—because it's not as sexy as get-rich-quick stories—is how the majority of rich people have built their wealth, using the values of time, patience, smarts, diversity, discipline, consistency, and generosity. While the work isn't always very exciting, it's a simple but proven formula that works every time. With good fortune added in or by placing calculated bets on opportunities when they appear without forcing it, we can end up with more than we'll ever need and more resources with which we can bless others.

I didn't learn these values all at once, and neither will you. The key is getting the basics down early, when you're leaving college or about to get your first job.

I had a mentor when I was getting ready to graduate from college who taught me to save two dollars out of every ten dollars I earned—to give one dollar away, invest the second, and then live off the other eight. He told me that money can make a person very happy, but it'll depend on what we do with it and whether we're in charge of it or it's in charge of us. "Work hard," he said, "be smart about applying the foundational values, and always remember to take off the top the two dollars out of every ten."

Time is a crucial factor in building wealth. The principles of asset growth and compounded interest are sound financial advice from down through the years. It's something you can easily do too. Consider these timeless principles of good money management:

- Live below your means; spend less than you earn.
- Pay yourself first; take 20 percent off the top.
- Invest 10 percent and give away 10 percent.
- Avoid bad debt, such as credit card balances and high-interest loans; home mortgage, transportation costs, and investments such as real estate can be good debt.
- Diversify investments and keep risk in check.
- Have patience; let time work its money magic.

The practical implications of adopting these principles means you'll take 20 percent off the top of every paycheck or dollar earned, without question, starting at a young age. Once you get used to it, you won't miss the 20 percent. It can be scary initially, but you'll quickly develop self-confidence in your future because you're investing your first 10 percent of your earnings and you'll have the satisfaction of helping others by donating 10 percent to organizations whose missions you believe in. (Keep in mind that you can get tax benefits from the contributions.)

It's not always what a man wants to hear: *Really? Save 10 percent and give away 10 percent of everything I make?* In my case, I chose to follow this strategy because I respected the man who mentored me, and I couldn't think of any better plan. I knew that stacking up money by investing for my own benefit the entire 20 percent I saved wouldn't get me anywhere. When asked how much money is enough, John D. Rockefeller, one of the world's richest men in his day, is said to have replied, "Just a little bit more."[13] Our accumulation of wealth will never seem enough, so I took my mentor's advice and gave 10 percent of my earnings to the church and other nonprofit organizations in my twenties.

Following this strategy wasn't easy, to be sure. When I was about to make my first-ever online charity donation, I entered the amount and had my credit card lined up to pay. All I had to do was hit submit. But my finger froze; it wouldn't hit the button. Finally, I counted to three, one to three . . . and click. Immediately, I felt not just okay but deeply satisfied because I knew I had earned money to support a cause I believed in.

The money I saved from the 10 percent didn't seem like much, and to be honest, it wasn't. But it began to add up. I invested in stocks that went up over time. Some years were better than others, but I tried not to overthink my strategies.

I made informed buys and tried to stay disciplined and trust the process because I learned that it's a winning strategy over time. I sometimes made risky bets based on my research and my feelings about my findings. I wasn't shooting from the hip. Some of these buys worked while some ended up in a total loss. But I had only allocated 30 percent of my stock investments into risky bets, while the other 70 percent went into time-tested blue chips. I kept other savings in a high-yield savings account or a certificate of deposit in case I needed it.

You'll notice a simple but important aspect of this strategy: I was in control. I made my money work for me instead of the other way around. Peace, comfort, pride, satisfaction, and happiness resulted because I took charge and made investment decisions based on sound information and a desire to make donations to benefit others.

Six years ago, in my early thirties, I knew it was time to diversify beyond stocks and savings. I had done enough research on friends who had invested in real estate. One of my friends had built a duplex to rent out, and it was clear it would be a strong investment. I wanted to get in on that.

To make my first real estate investment, I had to liquidate some of my stock holdings and withdraw some savings—funds I had grown comfortable having. But the move wasn't stupid; it was calculated. I was nervous, but I leaned on people for guidance who knew the market through its ups and downs.

When I closed on my first duplex, I knew I could clear

$1,000 a month over the banknote. I could increase my living expenses if I wanted to keep up with what I saw other guys my age doing, or I could double down on that investment and get another duplex. I opted for more real estate investments and soon found myself with multiple properties that were growing in value and delivering a steady income to pay off the banknote. I let my money work for me.

When it comes to giving, I learned that it's good to donate both large amounts of money, which often means writing out a check or making an online payment that doesn't result in personal engagement, and small amounts to nonprofits and individuals to address specific needs. I broke the grip that fear had on me about giving my money away. I became equipped to control money instead of allowing it to control me.

A student in one of my classes wanted to go on a mission trip but couldn't afford it. I wanted to pay his expenses but wanted to do it anonymously. After he came back from the trip, he told stories of his experiences with great excitement, his eyes wide with joy and his smile broad. I could see the impact it made, and it moved me as much as if I had gone on the trip myself. If I had told him I had helped him, it could have taken his joy away and caused him to feel as though he owed me something. I know he will one day pay it forward in his acts of generosity. That was enough for me because it was a gift to me as much as it was a gift to him.

By all means, pursue your financial goals. If wealth is your ambition for the right reasons, double down. Give it all you have. You are created to achieve, and I believe in you. But remember that achievement and money can't fix you.

And remember, too, that if all you can manage in your twenties and thirties is paying for essentials like rent and food, plus maybe something like a gym membership, while investing 10 percent and giving away 10 percent, this accomplishment has you on a path to more money and greater opportunities. You are just getting started, and you can't measure yourself against the earnings of your father, who worked a lifetime to get him to where he is today.

The desire for instant wealth is often rooted in a lack of self-esteem. Most financially successful men I meet didn't get there easily or quickly. It's abundantly clear that social media is misleading, and what you see around you can be misleading too. If wealth is meant for you, it will come, but only if you stop chasing riches and focus instead on the day in front of you and continue putting your plan into action.

You are in charge. Money is a tool. Let it work for you.

TIPS

- ➔ Remember, money won't make you a man, and money alone won't bring you joy. When you're pursuing a material goal like a new car or house, ask yourself, *What do I really want?* It may not be the actual thing, but rather what that thing can bring you. Understanding the root of your desire helps you determine whether or not to pursue it.
- ➔ Cultivating financial discipline in your twenties and thirties can help you achieve your goals. Invest and give, and you will receive in return.
- ➔ Building wealth and financial strength slowly and consis-

tently over time is always the best strategy. Get-rich-quick schemes are enticing but all too often result in failure.

→ Take a step back and think about what you can value above and beyond the endless pursuit of things.

13

SEX WON'T SAVE YOU

SEX WITHOUT LOVE IS AS HOLLOW AND RIDICULOUS AS LOVE WITHOUT SEX.

HUNTER S. THOMPSON, AUTHOR

If there's one area in which culture's messages to men are even more misleading than the messages about money, it's sex. So it's worth stating this clearly: Seeing sex as a competition, as a proving ground for manhood, diminishes our strength and character as men and harms our long-term satisfaction with sex and romantic relationships.

It is a cultural lie that growing the number of sexual partners will build us up as men. The truth is, doing so can break us or at the very least diminish us, making us feel bad about ourselves and inflicting similar harm on our partner.

That's why many Gen Zers are quietly stepping away from the hookup culture that dominated the previous generation. They're tired—tired of swiping through dating profiles, tired of sex without substance, tired of relationships without meaning. A recent study found that college students increasingly prefer to meet through real friendships, not dating apps built for instant gratification.[1]

Hookup culture hasn't disappeared though. As Americans wait longer to marry (nearly four years later on average than a generation ago), sex without commitment has become more normalized in working-class communities. And always lurking in the background is the body count bravado, the influence of porn, the curated lies of social media, and a rising tide of low self-worth.

What I'm saying isn't about judgment; it's about truth. You deserve more. And so does the person you're with.

The fact is that the more a guy relies on his sexual conquests, or body count, to boost his ego, the farther his self-esteem and satisfaction will fall—to say nothing of the human being with emotions who is on the other side of any encounter. (The phrase "body count" is taken from the context of war, where it refers to the number of people killed. If that doesn't reveal how dehumanizing and destructive this way of thinking is, I don't know what does.)

A study of 1,468 college students on the emotional aftermath of hookups found that about 83 percent of college students reported emotional harm after hookups—including feelings of embarrassment, loss of self-respect, and difficulty sustaining healthy relationships.[2] Another study revealed that around 78 percent of women and 72 percent of men felt regret after uncommitted sex.[3] While various studies differ in their conclusions, repeated casual encounters have been linked to higher rates of anxiety and depression, potentially fueling the adolescent mental health crisis.[4]

My discussions with college students reveal that their feelings mirror these statistics. They say they feel ashamed and frustrated with an abundance of casual sex and the pressure to make it seem like it's simply a stimulating activity that's easy to walk away from. The men in their twenties and thirties I work with say sex without strings makes them feel hollow and of precious little value.

Yet many men are keeping score, trying to boost their sagging self-esteem, using body count as a bragging point for themselves and among friends, while often condemning the same practice in women in a judgmental double standard.

Some guys put together an actual list. A few of my clients have shown me their lists on their phone's notes app; others keep a mental list. But here's a fundamental problem with the concept: Keeping score turns sex into an empty competition, meaning we end up with more meaningless hookups and fallout than we want or need. Yet many men continue to keep a tally in their minds and even share it with friends. They do so for these reasons:

- pride (ego boost and status among peers)
- validation (false evidence of your worth)
- immaturity (inability to see the human being on the other side)
- group competition (guys trying to outdo one another)

None of these are good reasons. Most hookups in the college years happen after substance use, a behavior that often continues beyond college. The problem is that hookups after heavy drinking often lead to guilt and shame and other ill-fated outcomes, including sexually transmitted diseases, physical consequences, and unwanted pregnancies. Consider also the phenomenon known as "catching feelings," where one party in a hookup that was supposed to be meaningless emerges with an *uh-oh, I kinda like you* feeling and ends up emotionally wounded.

Studies suggest a majority of men (and women) would be happier with one meaningful person and relationship. Take, for example, the study conducted by the National Bureau of Economic Research in which people with one sexual partner a year are happier than those with two or more.[5] Other research shows that casual sex is associated with "psychological distress, including anxiety and depression, as well as low self-esteem and reduced life satisfaction."[6]

Many other studies reveal that marriages in which both spouses had slept only with each other are more satisfied with their marriages, including having a greater degree of sexual and emotional closeness. In other words, less sexual experience before marriage equals greater satisfaction in marriage, according to the studies.[7]

TRYING TO FILL A VOID

In my own life, rejection was the thing I was trying to fix when it came to sex. My story started in college. I was nineteen and wasn't getting noticed by girls much. Then, when as

I mentioned earlier, a guy called me skinny, I started going to the gym, telling myself, *I'm never going to let that happen again*.

Anytime you put *never* in a statement, you aren't heading in the right direction. That's how it was for me in the gym. My goal was to lift enough to become good enough. *You call me ugly, and I'm going to do something about it.*

After several months of working out, I had gained five to ten pounds of muscle—enough to see a difference. I started carrying myself differently. The enhanced muscle and posture earned me attention in the gym I didn't get before.

Soon after, I had my first random hookup with a girl, which produced euphoria in the moment and emptiness immediately afterward. Drugs have never been my thing, but I've worked with enough people who have had that struggle, and let me tell you, what I began to battle was much the same. I got the hit of dopamine and euphoria through the hookup, and even though I didn't feel good afterward, I went back for more. The euphoria pulled me back like a drug.

I did it again and again.

It's a sex slope. When we step onto the top of the cliff by means of a hookup, it's thrilling in the moment. We jump, but we keep falling, and we can't really stop until we crash at the bottom.

The euphoria lessened each time. It was never the same as that first jolt. I still felt some thrill of the hunt and the pleasure of the sex itself, but *boom*, it was quickly over, and I was left feeling empty and alone. And so I kept running away from myself and toward the next fix—a vicious cycle on repeat. If you talk to anyone who struggles with substance use disorder, they'll tell you it's the same phenomenon.

Eventually, I realized I had trained my brain in these hookups to shut off feelings so there'd be no emotional connection. In the beginning, that was the point. Smooth sailing, get something for nothing. But it was a road to emptiness and shame.

I had a desire for connection, but I was still maturing emotionally. By going straight to the hookup, neither I nor the girl received any of the benefits of genuine connection. I trained my body to respond physically but not emotionally, and I developed an avoidant attachment style, with a strong desire for independence and a significant difficulty in trusting others.

If we don't take steps to break a negative pattern, that pattern can engulf us. I'd go on binge streaks of casual encounters until I recognized the damage I was doing and stopped. I would then try dating, but between my addiction to the quick-fix affirmation and the distrust of myself and the relationships I had developed, those relationships never worked.

I was experiencing a sad reality: If we are a train wreck ourselves, we'll never attract the right person. Whenever I thought, *Wow, this might be the right one*, I could feel myself holding back, which is exactly what I had trained myself to do.

I was looking for a connection but ended up with pain. All along, part of me knew I was digging myself into a hole, lying to myself to keep myself buried. I thought when I found the right girl, I'd stop. But I was hearing false affirmations from the women I hooked up with because they suffered just as I did. We were all there for the wrong reasons, telling ourselves and each other the same lie, and we slipped further away each time from the lives we were meant to live.

Eventually, I had enough. The first step with any addiction is admitting we have a problem. Then we must realize we can't do it alone, that it's bigger than we are. My addiction was certainly bigger than me, and I needed God, the support of friends, some good counseling, and new habits to make a change.

I'm thankful I didn't force myself into a relationship while I was working through all this. But I also reflect back on a couple women I dated who were the real deal, who could have been a lifetime partner, but I know now they could see I was only paying lip service to wanting a healthy relationship. I knew what to say, but I needed to work on escaping the hookup culture and building new habits so I could be ready when the right one came into my life.

PUSH BACK AGAINST THE PATTERN

On of the benefits I gained from my experience of sex addiction is that as I see it in many men I work with, I can better relate to and help them. I've been there. Many will come to the early sessions, throwing ego and bravado, bragging about body count and conquests.

They have become so accustomed to other men cheering or acting like they're achieving such great things, they think I'll be impressed. I listen, because that's my job. But they hear soon enough about the loneliness of that experience, and that can bring them face-to-face with the truth.

They've been taught that the only way to prove their masculinity is through sexual conquest, which they must do more than their friends. They feel that if they aren't having sex to brag about, they are a failure or something is wrong with them. But instead, they are lost and hollow and are in profound need of connection and relationship.

Shawn, in his early twenties, had had more sex than he could recall since beginning high school, yet he never actually dated anyone or had a serious girlfriend. He felt alone and unsatisfied with his life. When I asked him why he hadn't asked girls out in high school, he said it was a waste of time since "my hormones were raging and all I wanted to do was hook up." I asked him why he didn't date in college, and he said, "I'd have looked stupid, since nobody did it." I asked him what he really wanted.

He shrugged.

"It was all about hooking up," he said, "having some fun with as many girls as possible before I'd have to settle down."

Shawn was spending nights at home by himself because he hadn't developed the interpersonal dating skills needed to cultivate relationships. Most of the hookups he proudly viewed as conquests happened after nights of drinking, so he barely remembered them, and most of them hadn't involved much talk beyond whatever chatter occurred at the bar. These "conquests" weren't victories at all; they were losses that left him hollow. And the women he'd hooked up with were likely feeling similarly hollow, since studies reveal that women often feel ashamed and bad about themselves after hookups.[8]

Except for Shawn's drinking, I could relate. I found myself grimacing when he spoke because of the familiarity. I reminded him that I didn't judge him for his behavior and that I had been there. I then shared how I had altered my behavior.

I challenged Shawn to implement the "why" questioning of himself, to turn back the dial to figure out what landed him in the situation.

- *Why did I leave with another woman when I didn't want to? Because I was at the bar having drinks and couldn't say no.*
- *Why did I go to the bar? Because I was feeling lonely after work.*
- *Why am I feeling lonely after work? Because I've hooked up with so many women that I have developed a reputation and the ones I want to settle with won't give me a look.*

He found the answer himself. To get what he wants—a life with someone to grow with—the hookups had to stop. To stop the hookups, his visits to the bar had to stop. To stop visits to the bar, he needed to find something to do with his time after work.

"What hobbies do you enjoy?" I asked.

"Running," he said. "I ran cross-country in high school and still love it."

We identified his injury—the message that he wasn't good enough—and observed that sex was the way he was medicating. Then we began to heal the injury.

If you're keeping a body count—whether on paper or just in your head—it's time to think again. It's not just a number; it's a wound that cuts both ways. It hurts you, and it hurts the people you hook up with.

The truth? Hookups won't fill what's missing. They'll just leave you feeling emptier—sad, disconnected, craving something more but not sure what. You may not want to hear this, but I'm telling you because I care. Because I've lived it. And I'd rather help you avoid the pain than have you learn your lesson the hard way like I did.

Take back your power. Start by asking why: *Why am I chasing this? What am I really hoping to feel?*

When you begin to answer those questions honestly, you'll find the strength to shift your focus from conquest to connection, from distraction to depth. This is where you will find the greatest satisfaction in your movement toward connection.

TIPS

- → Talk out loud with someone you trust about the issues relating to sex. When we keep our feelings about sex in the dark, we are setting ourselves up to feeling stuck.
- → Ask yourself, *What benefit am I getting from hooking up besides feeling good in the moment?*
- → Ask yourself, *How might I feel after a hookup, and how might the other person feel?* (It will impact them too, even if they are consenting to it and want it.)
- → Visualize the marriage you want. Then do some reverse engineering to see what it'll take to achieve that.
- → What's your take on this question? *Will hookups push me closer to or farther from my goals regarding marriage?*

14

CHANGE YOUR BODY, CHANGE YOUR BRAIN

Your mind is a gift. It gives you thoughts, emotions, creativity, problem-solving skills, and the ability to make deep connections. It helps you feel both anger and empathy. But here's the truth: Your mind—your mental clarity, focus, and emotional regulation—can only reach its full potential when your body is strong and well cared for.

A strong, well-nourished body fuels a healthy, high-performing brain. Together, they fuel a stronger you. That's why ignoring your physical health isn't an option if you want to build real strength.

Your body—from brain and muscles to bones and blood flow—is a masterpiece. And it was made to work in harmony. This harmony between mind and body isn't accidental; it's built into your design. And for men, a key characteristic of that design is strength.

Testosterone fuels our strength. It's produced primarily by our testicles and is the difference between men and women. Women's bodies produce and circulate some testosterone, but healthy men from puberty have fifteen to twenty times more. It fuels our sex drive and builds our muscles while also enhancing mood and body fat distribution. Testosterone is one of our greatest assets as men, and we must protect it because it's vital fuel for a healthy body and mind. But testosterone levels can drop, even among young men, for a number of reasons, including being overweight, inactive, or sleep-deprived.

Alcohol and drug misuse or steroid use for bodybuilding are other reasons testosterone levels can drop in younger men. For most, it's a vicious cycle where testosterone levels drop due to a sedentary lifestyle, weight gain, and loss of quality sleep. Your mood drops along with it. Your anxiety increases, along with depression and mental fogginess. Your energy is low and you know you should work out, but you don't have the drive to do it. Your quality of life diminishes a little more month after month, year after year.

It's more than just low energy that keeps men from working out. Here's an official list of reasons provided by the US Centers for Disease Control and Prevention:

Reasons Adults Don't Exercise[1]

- lack of time
- lack of social support

- lack of energy
- lack of motivation
- fear of injury
- lack of skill
- high cost and lack of facilities
- weather conditions

Whatever the reason, however, it all comes down in the end to one thing—drive. If you have the will, you can cultivate the drive. Once you have the drive, you can push through the list of excuses to form new habits and transform your body and nourish your mind.

We discussed earlier how asking ourselves why can help address contextual excuses and remove obstacles that stand in the way of achieving our goals. We can apply the "why question" strategy to our excuses for not exercising.

Let's deal first with the issue of *time*. Take a look at each day over the past week. Do you see any open slots to squeeze in thirty minutes of exercise? Cut out streaming in the evening, scrolling social media, or gaming, and you may find you have the time you need. Do you feel a lack of support? Need some friends to encourage you on your journey? Share with others your desires and needs and ask if they have similar interests. I'll bet they do. When men get together with friends to work out, we can experience some of our best camaraderie.

Feeling low on energy? Start with jogging, climbing stairs, or swimming to get the blood flowing to your brain, boosting your energy level. If you aren't ready for that, try yoga or walking long distances at a brisk pace. Still putting it off? Avoid taking the easy way out. Do you have stairs at your office building? Climb them. Are you paying someone to do yard work or household chores? Do them yourself.

All physical activity sends blood to our brain, immediately improving mood and decreasing feelings of anxiety, depression, or stress.[2] It's not just about our mind or our testosterone levels, though those are reasons enough. Exercise improves blood flow, which is key for arousal in sex. That means more exercise equals better sex.[3] Men who don't work out, who aren't physically fit, face higher rates of cardiovascular disease, obesity, high blood pressure and cholesterol, diabetes, stroke, and cancer.[4] These aren't things younger men typically think about. We can take arousal and physical health for granted because it happens easily. We may think nothing of eating a plateful of fries and fried chicken four days in a row with no exercise because we feel invincible. But take that behavior into our middle-aged years, and it doesn't turn out so well.

Look at it this way: We get just one body, which we should take care of at every age as we strive to develop strength and fitness. Theodore Roosevelt provides a good example. Regarded as one of the most successful presidents in United States history (1901–1909), Roosevelt was a sickly child with asthma who slouched and was susceptible to attacks by bullies. Roosevelt's father said, "Theodore, you have the mind, but you have not the body; and without the help of the body the mind cannot go as far as it should. I am giving you the tools, but it is up to you to make your own body."[5]

Roosevelt listened to his father and took up boxing as a young man, and engaged in tennis, swimming, weight lifting, hiking, polo, and other sports and physical activities throughout his life. He became a fitness fanatic who advocated for "the strenuous life." Roosevelt believed that "in this life we get nothing save by effort," that upholding one's moral and physical character is in essence a patriotic duty.[6] Today we still have that duty—to ourselves, our family and friends, and our community—to be our best with a healthy body and mind.

"Exercise till the mind feels delight in reposing from the fatigue," said Socrates, the Greek philosopher who died in the year 399 BC.[7] Still, only about 25 percent of adults in the United States meet the government's Physical Activity Guidelines for both weekly aerobic and muscle-building activities. The recommendations are at least 150 minutes to 300 minutes of moderate-intensity exercise or 75 to 150 minutes of vigorous-intensity aerobic exercise per week, with additional muscle-strengthening activities such as weight-lifting of moderate or greater intensity two days a week for maximum healthy benefits. More men than women meet the aerobic recommendations, but many don't also add in muscle strengthening, which means there's a lot of opportunity for life improvement.[8]

THE RIGHT REASONS

I talked earlier about what got me into the gym initially and what kept me going back. It began with my ego and weakness, but as my body grew stronger, I began to think more clearly. I had time at the gym to ask myself why.

I began to realize that a stronger body gave me more

confidence. And it wasn't about being attractive to women; it was about being a man—being strong enough to recognize my weaknesses. I loved how working out allowed me to set goals and push through discomfort to meet or exceed them. I loved how working out helped alleviate the anxiety and pressure I faced outside of the gym. I loved how it strengthened both my body and my mind and gave me confidence that I could contribute with my strength through my hard work.

I started small, stacking little wins and building momentum. I recommend this approach for everyone. Don't try to do too much at once, but don't doubt what you can achieve either. All of us can carry more weight than we expect, which is why weight lifting and aerobic exercise is a great lesson and metaphor for life. What looks hard becomes easier once we do the work. The type of exercise will vary from person to person. You may not enjoy weight lifting. Perhaps you prefer bicycling, hiking mountain trails, or doing yoga.

Ole Miss football coach Lane Kiffin quit drinking alcohol not long after COVID-19 because he saw that it wasn't providing any benefit. "I didn't hit a rock bottom," he said, "I just got tired. Tired of digging myself out of messes I would create."[9] He found the strength to quit drinking by deepening his faith and by doing yoga and engaging in other physical activity multiple days a week. Some days, Oxford, Mississippi, residents saw him in a hot yoga class early in the morning and a Pilates class later in the day. On game days, he took a private yoga class or had staff members join with him.

Kiffin's body was transformed—you can see the difference in the images over the years—and his mind and emotions benefited as well. He said he is better able to handle the intense stress of his coaching and recruiting duties while being thankful for his gifts of family and community.

The mental health benefits of physical activity can be enjoyed by everyone. A study of 1.2 million US adults from various demographic backgrounds showed that those who exercised had better mental health functioning compared to nonexercisers.[10] Bettering your body to better your mind is like making a guaranteed investment for easy money. You make deposits with regular exercise and get riches of improved mental health as dividends. Here are some of them:

- mood enhancement (regular exercise has benefits similar to those of antidepressant medications)
- increased confidence
- enhanced community building and engagement
- increased energy and testosterone
- strengthened muscles and bones
- improved sex life
- better overall health and lifespan
- healthier brain and memory

Making changes to your body is not just about working out; it's also about what you put into your body. Feed the caveman with more protein and less processed foods and keep everything in moderation. Also remember the importance of regeneration and practice it consistently. Our bodies were built to recover, which means we don't function well without rest. Most healthy men need seven to nine hours of sleep a night. The amount may vary for individuals, but less than seven hours on a consistent basis is unhealthy. Even one day with too little sleep can leave us irritable, less able to focus, low on energy, and down in mood. Our diet and rest patterns are as important as working out, but for me, it begins with exercise because physical activity leads to better eating and sleeping.

Consider a study by researchers at the University of Texas that found young adults who were once sedentary and then added exercise for several weeks selected better food choices without instruction.[11] Another study showed that young people who exercise sleep longer and better.[12] Just being sedentary for one day can interrupt our sleep and diet, while being active for one day can have an immediate positive impact.

You know this anecdotally, of course. Go for a long run, and you feel invigorated and healthy, and you're apt to avoid the fried food platter for dinner. No sense wasting all that effort you put into your exercise. Later, you'll sleep long and deep that night—your best night's sleep in weeks. But sit around the house most of the day, and you're more likely to down the bag of chips you intended to avoid and stay up late streaming a movie, even though you have to get up early the next morning. When you're not rested, your body and mind suffer. You may exhibit signs of ADHD with accompanying fatigue, mood swings, and irritability.

When I'm working with high school students, I can tell the minute a young person walks into the room if they haven't had enough sleep. One guy showed up angry with a scowl. Everything he said was negative. So I asked him, "How much sleep are you getting?"

The question annoyed him. "I don't need much sleep," he

said, as he went on to tell me about all the As he was getting at school.

"How much is not much?"

"Well, I slept three hours last night. That's about normal."

"Three hours!"

I explained the science about sleep requirements, and he smirked.

I and asked him to do me a favor—to prove me wrong by getting seven or eight hours for several nights and then come back to see me. He responded, "I'm not gonna be able to get to sleep," so I asked him what kind of exercise he liked.

"I used to like running," he said.

"Go out and run several miles first thing in the morning and see what happens."

A few days later, he came back a different person.

"I'm sorry," he said. "I was strung out from so little sleep, and I couldn't think straight."

He told me about his running and that he was making plans for the weekend with friends—talking in an almost awe-struck voice like he had come back to life, all because he had been jogging a couple miles each day and getting seven or more hours of sleep.

It reminded me of a story about the SEC commissioner Greg Sankey. As the leader of one of the most successful sports leagues in the world, collegiate or professional, Sankey is under a lot of performance pressure. When the United States shut down for COVID-19 in 2020, everyone wondered what would come next. There was talk that college sports would never be the same.

Sankey didn't have the answers, and he felt the stress as

people died and uncertainty lingered. Everything was shut down, including the gym where he worked out. Sankey decided to take charge of his destiny. He took off from his house in Birmingham, Alabama, and went running for thirty-five minutes. Every day thereafter, for a couple years, Sankey ran for at least thirty-five minutes, losing thirty pounds and four inches from his waist. He credited running with helping him make difficult decisions during the pandemic, such as when to allow student athletes back to campus for workouts.

"It was just great mental therapy for me, and given what we were dealing with, I said, 'I'm going to go for a run,'" Sankey said. "That's really how it started, was a recognition of, I needed to do something."[13]

Do something. We all have the power to do something. I do. You do. Don't delay. Do something—today. Strengthen your body and sharpen your mind. Just imagine what you can do when you resolve to get going on the journey toward a stronger body and mind. If you aren't working out, it's time. If you have a routine, take it to the next level or add another challenge that keeps it refreshing and enjoyable.

Remember, we are wired for strength. We flourish when we nurture and hone that strength. When we make change in our bodies and minds, we change our lives in the process.

YOU ARE BUILT FOR THIS

The key for anyone who is just starting out is not to get overwhelmed. Start with something you enjoy and set achievable goals. Don't waste time envying someone who goes to the gym multiple days a week and has the pecs and biceps that come from years of work. Start small, setting goals that increase over time. As you become stronger and add endurance, track these goals.

When we set goals, we have better odds of both achieving and continuing on, because we can track progress and see the fruits of our labor. Celebrate milestones, sharing them with friends and family who show interest in your growth. Celebrate the bigger ones the same way you would a birthday. Birthdays are worth celebrating, and everyone gets to have one. However, not everyone can push themselves toward establishing and pursuing their goals. Celebrate your victories!

Don't be afraid to push yourself either. We possess far more physical capacity than we think we do, especially as we're starting out. By avoiding discomfort, we avoid our potential. I've watched men who struggled to bench press one hundred pounds go on to triple their strength and drop their body fat in less than a year. When we remove distractions, set goals, and push through discomfort, what once felt impossible becomes achievable. If we can push ourselves to another mile or set our sights on bench pressing that heavier weight, we can better handle what life throws at us. If we dread the extra weight, we are more likely to struggle against the hard in life.

A friend of mine who thrives on pushing through discomfort worked out at the same gym as his sister's boyfriend. He couldn't help but notice that the guy had a pattern. Every time the weight got too heavy or the strain too intense, the boyfriend backed off and quit. My friend eventually told his sister, "Hey, I'm worried that this guy isn't the one for you.

From what I see, when things get tough, he's not going to be there for you."

My friend's sister didn't listen, but three weeks later, she came back to her brother and said, "You were right; he's not the guy. How did you know?"

I don't tell the story to say that the boyfriend was weak. He was very likely trying to find his strength. He liked the idea of going to the gym and working out, but it seemed that he hadn't yet set goals and benefited from the push. Maybe he'll get there.

The point is, fatigue feeds fatigue, and energy feeds energy.

When you work out and push yourself, you have more drive. Avoid the push, and you may well find yourself avoiding other hard things.

What activities will you do to invest in your body and mind? Ask yourself, *What am I more willing and likely to do and keep doing?* If you aren't sure, explore different things, including trying something new. It could be one of any number of activities—running, climbing, hiking, bicycling, power yoga, weight lifting, or Pilates. Each of us has different strengths and natural giftedness. The key is discovering what keeps us coming back for more, since *not* doing something is not an option.

Get in shape, and you'll feel better mentally and physically. You'll look better, and you'll think better—almost immediately.

In the end, it's all about finding what's right for you and learning to push through discomfort to get the reward.

TIPS

→ Commit to one easy habit you can consistently carry out, such as going to the gym with a fitness plan or establishing a regular pattern of running or biking. If you're already working out, add something new to keep it interesting.

- → Set achievable goals, say them out loud to yourself and someone else, and celebrate milestones in victory.
- → Find friends or a community to engage with, celebrate their achievements, and listen to their challenges.
- → Remember that you are positively shaping both your mind and your body. During workouts, embrace thoughts about your life as you currently experience it, your work, and your family and how you can be stronger in all of these aspects.

15

DISCIPLINE

WE ANSWER HUNDREDS OF QUESTIONS EVERY DAY THAT COME DOWN TO THESE TWO THINGS: HERE'S SOMETHING YOU KNOW YOU'RE SUPPOSED TO DO THAT YOU REALLY DON'T WANT TO DO. CAN YOU MAKE YOURSELF DO IT? AND THEN OVER HERE THERE'S SOMETHING YOU KNOW YOU'RE NOT SUPPOSED TO DO, BUT YOU WANT TO DO IT. CAN YOU KEEP YOURSELF FROM IT?

NICK SABAN, LEGENDARY ALABAMA COACH

Discipline is essential on the journey to becoming a man of genuine strength. It's one of our most important attributes because without it, we're vulnerable to distraction, self-doubt, comparison, temptation, and the constant pull to chase things that don't truly matter.

With discipline, we say no and mean it.

We keep pushing when we want to quit because we've made a commitment.

We hold our tongue when anger flares because we know restraint is stronger than reaction.

We skip the purchase we don't need because we're focused on what matters in the long term.

Think back on everything we've covered so far, especially distraction. We can't overcome it without discipline. The same goes for building our team, owning our decisions, standing up for ourselves, or making our money work for us. Every step of this journey requires discipline because real growth doesn't happen overnight. It's not a flip of a switch. It's a daily decision.

Discipline is learning to lead yourself. It's what keeps you on the path from where you are to where you want to be. Discipline is mindset—your practiced belief in who you are and what you're capable of. It's staying focused on the big goal while making the right small choices repeatedly. Think of it like this: Discipline is throwing pennies in a jar every day. It may not look like much, but one day you'll look back and see that the jar is full. You stayed the course. You became the man you set out to be.

Former New York Yankees star Derek Jeter provides a good example of a man of discipline. He was one of the greatest baseball players ever, a strong-hitting shortstop with talent, drive, and focus to match his flair on the diamond in the Big Apple.

He earned his success, spanning twenty years with the Yankees, because he felt like he "had to earn the right to play." Even though he was one of the game's best players, Jeter was known to go back to work within three to four weeks after one grueling season ended to prepare for the next, while many other players were enjoying a long break from training. He was working out, taking batting practice and fielding ground balls. "I've always felt as though, for me to do my job, I had to be disciplined." Jeter said.[1] This was Jeter following through on the vision he had of himself in elementary school, telling classmates in the fourth grade that he planned to play shortstop for the Yankees one day.

Without discipline, achieving that goal wouldn't have happened for Jeter. Without discipline, the vision doesn't happen for any of us.

The vast majority of us won't become a professional athlete, much less one of the greatest players ever in our particular sport. Still, with discipline, we can become all we are meant and want to be because we are consistently optimizing our performance when measured against our goals and expectations and gaining great results.

Discipline produces many benefits, such as the following:

- productivity
- strengthened willpower (consistently making the best choices for our future with discipline, which strengthens our neural pathways and builds new habits)
- self-power (internal validation over external validation)
- a focus on life's purpose (prioritizing what matters over chasing things for pleasure)

- taking responsibility (no more playing the blamc game)
- becoming the person you want to be

I mentioned earlier my eight-hour walk on a Saturday to discover what was bugging me. I wanted to quit about fifty times, but it was discipline that got me through. I think, too, about the time I committed to help crack a human trafficking case but was afraid I was getting in over my head once I got there.

I didn't naturally have the discipline needed for those moments and others I've faced. I had to develop it and cultivate it, just as everyone does. But practice makes us stronger. Instead of saying to ourselves, *No, I can't do that*, we say, *Yes, I can*. Discipline is a key to better managing all that life throws at us. Once we learn to say no to what brings us down and yes to what builds us up, discipline becomes enjoyable—a source of personal pride and strength that sets us apart, our secret weapon that guides us to positive change and clearer purpose.

Let's say you decide to run three days a week to meet the cardio recommendations for a healthy body. Don't just vaguely commit to it; plan it. Choose your days, your time of day, and your distance. Be specific. Details and consistency derail excuses before they can even get started.

When it's time to run, say a clear yes to yourself—for the energy, the confidence, the long-term health benefits. And when your mind tries to offer excuses—*I was up late*, or *my in-laws are in town*—respond with a firm, disciplined no. Shut that voice down. And get up and go.

Everyone has goals. Everyone dreams of being better. But not everyone has discipline. Be different. Be stronger.

When we practice discipline, it's like making steady deposits in our own success bank, and the return is exponential. Discipline gives us momentum. It aligns our actions with our values, character, and vision, an alignment that builds freedom, power, and confidence. When we live with discipline, nothing and nobody can hold us back—not even ourselves.

LOOK AT YOURSELF IN THE FUTURE

To gain the strength for discipline, it's helpful to look ahead. Ask yourself, *What's next for me?* By looking ahead, you give yourself the power to set clear goals and personal standards. You stop reacting and start leading. You solve problems before they start and become strong enough to face anything that comes your way.

Picture the future version of you—the one you admire and respect, the one who made peace with the past and grew stronger because of it, the one who is happiest, most fulfilled, and living with purpose. That version of you exists. But only if you're willing to envision it and work for it, with the focus, discipline, and commitment it takes to stay the course. The future you see and want is shaped by what you're willing to do today.

Envisioning your future self helps shift your perspective of your current situation. Studies show that negative perceptions can cause anxiety and depression and diminish overall well-being, while positive perceptions improve self-esteem and happiness while reducing anxiety and stress.[2]

Take, for example, being unhappy and unfulfilled at your job. It's likely we've all been there or will be there at some point in our career. Maybe you don't get along with your boss or coworkers, or you've concluded that you won't last long there or that it's a dead-end career. All you can think about is quitting, which makes you feel frustrated and depressed. Your anxiety grows daily, but you feel stuck, unsure of what to do, and you need the paycheck so you can't quit. Not yet.

When you feel stuck, chances are, you are focusing on the past. You ruminate about everything that has been done to you and hasn't happened for you. You analyze previous achievements and view with regret the decision that brought you to where you are in life.

But here's what seeing yourself in the future and practicing discipline will do for you: Imagine yourself in the job, the career, you want. Think about the life experience and characteristics that will help you land this opportunity. Now look at your current job and return to it with the discipline to work on areas that can help you achieve the future you envision. Quitting is easy, but growing, while more difficult, is far more productive.

Discipline helps you emerge stronger for your current job and better prepares you to seize the opportunities you want and deserve.

THE POWER OF POSSIBILITY

Too often, the young men I counsel struggle because they feel trapped by everything they are not. In other words, they don't feel like they are enough. They didn't become the college star quarterback who made it into the NFL draft. They didn't become the conductor of the symphony. They didn't become the valedictorian of their class. They didn't get the girl they dreamed of getting.

Josh fit the description of great expectations and dashed dreams. He was an all-stater in football in high school and a four-star recruit at wide receiver. Throughout high school and into college, he garnered all the attention, and classmates talked about how they were planning to see him in the NFL one day. But he and the coaching staff didn't click at his first school. He transferred for his sophomore year, even though his NIL money didn't increase. Then during his first game of the season, he got a concussion from a hit that left him wobbly on the field.

Josh had already suffered several concussions in high school, and the team doctor said he should seriously consider giving up football. But Josh was determined to get to the NFL. He got a special helmet that was supposed to reduce concussions.

Josh told me he saw football as his future and didn't know what else to do, so he kept playing, even after his sophomore-year concussion.

"It's all I've got," he said.

I smiled. "That's not all you've got," I said.

Josh was a tall kid with a big smile. He walked into the room, and everybody lit up. He was a natural leader who people wanted to get around and follow. On the team, he was considered another coach of sorts, giving tips and delivering uplifting messages to teammates.

Josh's natural charisma had nothing to do with football. If he lived in a different era when football wasn't a thing, he still would have stood out. But Josh believed that his worth was tied to his football accomplishments.

Late in his sophomore year, Josh got back into action. His second game back, he attempted a diving catch across the middle of the field, moving in the same direction as a cornerback coming in to try to knock the ball loose—and crack! Josh blacked out. He was stretched out on the field, out cold. It was the last football play he would ever participate in.

My work with Josh grew in intensity the next year because he firmly believed that at the age of twenty-one, his life and value was done.

I asked Josh what he loved.

"God, my family, and other people," he said.

"You didn't say football."

He smiled. "Naw, not first. That was just my thing. I loved the attention football gave me."

Josh said he enjoyed people, and his leadership inspired people to follow him. He ended up going into sales and thriving because he had a personality that everyone gravitated toward. Had he limped into his sales career, feeling like he failed in football, Josh would have struggled. When football ended, he initially felt like there was nothing left. He was at risk of becoming distracted, of sinking instead of rising in that moment of challenge.

We talked about the discipline he employed to excel in football—long, hot summers of lifting weights, and hours of practice while his friends were hanging out. That discipline, combined with his people skills, helped guide him to his future self. His self-esteem wasn't at the top when he began sales training, but he worked at it like he did at football, arriving early, staying late to ask questions in training. Today, he's winning at the thing he was meant to do.

There's always a tomorrow better than the hard today. Seeing ourselves in that tomorrow, and doing the work to get there, deliver the result.

Whenever you feel stuck, like Josh or the person who is miserable in their job and ready to quit without a plan, remember that you are not stuck. You hold the power to move and to keep moving.

Take a moment to look ahead to where you want to be in one year, or five years, and perhaps for many years to come. Imagine yourself doing work that will give you fulfillment and joy; imagine where and with whom you will live and what you'd like to do with your leisure, money, and time—living life as your best self. If you can picture it, you can set goals that can help you get there. With discipline, you can reach the goals and enjoy success.

This isn't just motivation talk. I see it in my life and in the lives of many men I counsel, and studies show that with discipline you are far more likely to become your best self—emotionally stronger and with a better attitude, qualities that lead to better jobs and relationships and greater fulfillment.[3]

TIPS

→ Think about the characteristics you admire in a strong and well-respected man and imagine yourself having those characteristics.

- → Spend quiet time envisioning yourself in the future as your best self. Imagine or draw a literal map that plots the way to get there. Revise your migration map as needed along the way.
- → Practice strengthening your discipline by setting specific, achievable goals and giving yourself strong noes and yeses in response as needed to stick to the goals.

16

HONED, CULTIVATED, AND FORGED

THE BEST WAY TO PREDICT THE FUTURE IS TO INVENT IT.

ALAN KAY, AMERICAN COMPUTER SCIENTIST

True leaders emerge when they discover something greater than ambition.

Everyone needs a battle worth giving their life to. You were born to do something meaningful with yours. This journey we're on, the path toward becoming strong enough to live your best life, is all about finding that meaning. It's about gaining the clarity, freedom, and strength to identify your purpose. Your why. The reason you get up every day. The reason you keep going when everything around you is hard. It's about aligning your daily actions with a greater mission and building the toughness to stay the course, no matter what comes your way.

Maybe you'll become one of the rare few whose impact is widely felt—like the doctor who cures childhood cancer after losing their own child or the quarterback who uses his financial success to lift families out of poverty because he himself came from a poor family. But the vast majority of us won't live on a public stage.

Still, that doesn't make your purpose any less important. When you help one person, you help many. The quiet strength of showing up, doing the work, and making someone else's life better—that's leadership. And that's a life of real meaning and incredible fulfillment.

HELPING ONE

The story of the starfish is a timeless parable about how making a difference even in small ways matters. The story is loosely based on Loren Eiseley's *The Star Thrower*, and it goes like this: A man was walking along a beach covered in thousands of stranded starfish. Looking up ahead, the man saw a young boy picking up one starfish after another and throwing them back into the ocean so they wouldn't die on the beach.

"But don't you realize that there are miles and miles of beach and starfish all along it," the man said. "You can't possibly make a difference!"

The young man bent down, picked up another starfish, and threw it into the ocean. "It made a difference for that one," he said.[1]

Indeed it did.

The one person we help may well pay it forward, and in turn that person may pay it forward as well, multiplying our efforts many times over, like the five loaves and two fish in Jesus' feeding of the five thousand (Matthew 14:13–21).

Just about everyone wants a sense of purpose. The challenge comes when we are bound by burdens, clouded by the wrong pursuits, and isolated from others. In these situations, we struggle to identify our gifts and passions, much less understand how to apply them. But as we do the work along this "tough enough" journey, we are poised and ready to discover our purpose and seize it with vigor, receiving all the due rewards along the way.

Having a sense of purpose is vital to our well-being and even our longevity. Studies show that with purpose, we can be healthier, sleep better, live longer, be happier and even make more money and have higher net worth.[2] Helping even just one person benefits both our well-being and that of the person we helped.

That's what they don't always tell you on those get-rich-quick videos—that by taking the long-road approach to life, odds are high that you *will* have it all. That doesn't mean life won't be hard. It certainly will. Hardship comes to everyone at one time or another, and for some people, adversity seems to hit more frequently and more severely. But you have the tools for resilience to navigate challenges and grow in pursuit of the goal to make a difference along the way.

CELEBRATE RECOVERY

Consider the story of the late pastor John Baker and his wife, Cheryl, of Saddleback Church in California. The year was 1991, and John, a member of the church staff, was in recovery and a participant in the twelve-step program Alcoholics Anonymous. Many in substance recovery have done exceptional self-work. By asking themselves why, turning to a higher power, and making peace with their past, they have cultivated a genuine strength that calls them to be like the boy who threw one starfish after another into the water without being overwhelmed by the reality that they can't help all the stranded starfish at once.

John Baker was the boy with the starfish when he went to Saddleback's senior pastor Rick Warren to tell him that he wanted to start a Christ-centered ministry for people in recovery, where they could "find freedom from their hurts, hang-ups, and habits."[3]

At the first meeting, forty-three people came—a big number, but small in comparison of what was to come. But the only initial ambition was serving those forty-three people.

It was the beginning of the Celebrate Recovery movement for men and women. Among the first people saved by the program was Johnny Baker, the son of Pastor John and his wife, Cheryl. Today, Johnny, in recovery as an alcoholic, leads Celebrate Recovery with his wife, Jeni, to global impact, serving within more than 35,000 churches and helping more than five million people.

The movement didn't start chasing the goal of global impact. It began at one church because the life of a pastor and his wife were changed by God and fellowship in recovery, and they wanted to help others within their community. That first forty-three turned into five million because they built the movement upon a foundation of genuine strength.

Even if substance misuse or addiction isn't something you've struggled with, you are entering into a phase of recovery and growth as a man because you, too, are doing the work to identify injuries, heal, take responsibility, and serve. We all have something to recover from—maybe overspending, self-absorption or a lack of self-confidence—and we all have areas for growth.

Remember, recovery doesn't always mean overcoming something dramatic or awful. Recovery happens when as people change, they improve their health and well-being so they can begin to live a life they take charge of and reach their full potential.

What does recovery mean?

- Recovery means growth—honing, cultivating, and forging.
- Recovery means learning to live life more freely and powerfully, despite what comes your way, despite those who try to bring you down.

- Recovery means rebuilding and regaining the innate strength you were given—a strength that the world and its culture and narratives try to steal from you.
- Recovery means you are stronger than before, tough enough to see and seize the path on which you belong, the place where you can make the most difference.
- Recovery means you can better discover your passion and purpose for life with peace and resiliency.
- Recovery means you can concentrate on positively impacting people's lives, not trying to impress them.
- Recovery means you attract followers and friends naturally.
- Recovery means you pursue work and life for the right reasons.
- Recovery means you aren't perfect. We are human beings. We are imperfect. And that's why we need one another, why we need discipline, why we need faith in a higher power.

Distraction will chase you throughout your life. So will people who don't have your best interests in mind and a world that doesn't care if you lose sight of your purpose. But you have what it takes to begin that journey today and never look back—recovering from injury and growing stronger as a man enroute to finding and living out your purpose. That's why you must peel those layers that hold you back so you can hone habits and forge a genuine strength that endures.

Understanding that you are on a journey alleviates the pressure to find and declare a purpose immediately, because your path of purpose is revealed in its time, when you are ready. By asking better questions of yourself, you can better find your path. For example, instead of asking, *What's my purpose?*—that's overwhelming—ask instead, *How can I be useful right now?* You'll experiment, learn, grow, and pursue the vision that serves as your North Star.

Some Important Questions to Ask Yourself That Can Guide You in Your Journey

- *If money were no object, how would I spend my time?*
- *As I look back over recent years, when did I feel most fulfilled?*
- *What are my strengths and talents?*
- *When others seek my counsel, what is it typically about?*
- *What do I want to change about the world or my community?*

The basic formula is **passion plus service equals purpose**.

Explore your passions, your job, and your goals with curiosity, and remember that you can and likely will revise these things along the way. We all change throughout life, and our passions and abilities change. Revision allows us to grow and shift without apology and overthinking.

I have a friend who is good with engines and working with his hands. He was energized by repairing people's vehicles and getting them back into service. He thrived on more complex jobs, such as repairing the older cars owned by clients who were struggling to make ends meet. He took great satisfaction from knowing his labor was helping them. Then after several years, he grew weary of his job. Cars had become more computerized, and small shops like his were facing obstacles. He lost his passion for that job but transitioned to woodworking, bringing to it the same passion for working with his hands and using his creativity to bless others with good things.

It's worth noting that my friend was quite successful in both of his businesses. An artisan, his work commanded a premium. Look around, and you'll see that almost everyone you identify as having a purpose has a corresponding experience of success. It's ironic that when we are aimless and chasing money and things, it's nearly impossible to get them, except for the rare few who get lucky—and even then, it's not truly lucky because they will struggle with success because they have a shaky foundation.

Do the right thing for the right reason with a strong foundation in place, and good fortune visits you because you've stacked the odds in your favor. Purpose gives you the strength to walk away from those who don't have your best interests at heart. Purpose keeps you grounded, focused, motivated, and equipped to handle whatever life throws at you. You no longer have to chase opportunities. Instead, they will find you, allowing you to pick and choose with strength and discipline.

The past got you to this point. It shaped and influenced you, and you navigated, learned, and arrived at the now. And you are ready now to step into the next phase, the most rewarding yet—because you are tough enough to grow and thrive beyond what you have known and experienced. You are ready for all that is to come, for all that you earn—including self-respect, the respect of others, and all the rewards that come with that.

A man of genuine strength and purpose wakes up each day knowing who he is and why he is here. Some days will be harder than others—that's life. But his strength doesn't fade. He is prepared. He is resilient. He is rooted in purpose and finds joy in the mission. He seeks long-term peace, not short-term escape. He puts his mind and body in position to grow, to serve, and to thrive.

That man is you.

You are tough enough to love and lead—not just yourself, but others. You have the power to make a positive, lasting difference in this world. No one can do it for you. Not me. Not anyone. It's your choice. And it's your commitment.

So ask yourself, *What do I want my life to stand for? What do I want people to say about me when I'm gone?*

Take time to reflect on these questions and let the answers guide you. And when you stay the course, with discipline and purpose, you will cultivate the strength needed to live the life you were made for.

You are tough enough to thrive. And the world needs all of what only you can give.

TIPS

- → Think about the legacy you want to leave, the difference you want to make through your life. Ask yourself, *What do I want my life to count for? How do I want people to remember me?*
- → Begin now to shape your life around the purpose that is growing within you. Even when hardships come, stay focused on the character you are committed to building and the impact for good that you want to make.

ACKNOWLEDGMENTS

I'm thankful to the Zondervan team for believing in *Tough Enough* and for their passion for helping young men grow. Daniel Marrs, vice president and publisher, and Webster Younce, vice president and executive editor at Zondervan, sold me in our first conversation. I'm thankful for their efforts to see the book through.

Others who had a role in bringing this book to publication include friend and bestselling author David Magee. He suggested I had a book in me that could help young men, and he introduced me to his literary agent, Esmond Harmsworth, president of Aevitas Creative Management. Tragically, Esmond died of natural causes on April 9, 2025. I'm thankful for his role in bringing the manuscript to Zondervan.

It's also important to mention two men who played an important role in my life. I sincerely appreciate Lee Burns, head of school at McCallie School in Chattanooga, Tennessee. Lee champions and enthusiastically supports my work of helping young men grow healthy and strong. My longtime friend and mentor Kenny Sholl of McCallie School encouraged me to pursue a career in counseling. He saw in me what I had not yet seen in myself. I'm thankful for that and so much more.

APPENDIX

TIPS FOR BECOMING TOUGH ENOUGH

TIPS FOR KILLING DISTRACTION

→ Right now, give your brain sixty seconds of silence. Just be still and let it rest.

→ Next, notice what your brain wanted you to do to escape the silence. If our brains aren't used to silence, they'll look for a way out of it because our brains crave what's familiar.

→ Tomorrow, increase this time to ninety seconds, then add thirty seconds each day.

TIPS FOR RUNNING THROUGH DISCOMFORT

- → Remember a time when you made it through something hard. Today, feel the pride you felt then. Feel the strength you felt then.
- → Visualize what you want—a goal, an outcome, or anything you want to accomplish. Create as clear a picture of it as you can. Step into that scene, imagining yourself in a movie. Use that visualization as your power when the steps required to accomplish your goal get hard.
- → Figure out one small first step you could take toward the goal. It should be a little uncomfortable but not intense. Use your vision of what you want as your superpower to take that small first step.

TIPS FOR FINDING YOUR INJURIES

- → Think about your childhood and ask yourself:
  - *Does it make me feel sad or lonely when I remember my growing-up years?*
  - *Do I have a history of unhealthy relationships with food, substances like alcohol and marijuana, people, or all of the above and more?*
  - *How does it feel to be rejected?*
  - *What are my behavior patterns?*
  - *Do I feel different than others and misunderstood by others?*
  - *What in my life isn't going as I want it to? Who might be holding me back?*

TIPS FOR DRAFTING YOUR TEAM

- → Look at the people you spend most of your time with and ask, *Do they have my best interests at heart? Do they care about my growth and well-being?*
- → Make a list of values you respect, such as being trustworthy and being respectful to others. Ask yourself, *Do those around me hold these values?*
- → Seek team members who support your goals and who have goals you can support.
- → Be willing to learn and listen to an insultant who has your best interests at heart.
- → Keep your eyes open for mentors you can trust and learn from; be willing to mentor others as well.
- → Work on your interpersonal communication skills, including the ways you present yourself to and acknowledge others.

TIPS FOR ASKING YOURSELF WHY

- → Define a specific problem you feel bad about and look for some moments of quiet and alone time—on a walk, doing a workout, or driving in the car without music—and ask yourself why you're feeling bad about it.
- → Don't be afraid to ask yourself questions about your beliefs, morals, and motivations.
- → Ask yourself, *What do I want?*
- → Ask yourself, *Why do I stumble to get there?*
- → Make notes or journal entries so you have your answers right in front of you.

TIPS FOR GETTING TO KNOW YOUR CAVEMAN

→ Here's how to tell your inner caveman to calm down:
  - Touch your thumb to your first finger. Now touch your second finger. Now the third, then the fourth.
  - Next, do it in backward order.
  - Now touch each finger in random order.
  - Do it again, and this time speed it up.
  - Do it another time, but slower.
  - Finally, do it again in random order, and now say out loud the number of the finger you're touching. So "one" for the first finger, and so on.

→ Here's another way to tell the caveman to calm down:
  - Place your hand over the middle of your chest, near your heart.
  - Leave it there for two minutes.
  - This position can activate the same part of your brain as when you get a hug. It'll release endorphins that send "relax" signals to the caveman and boost your mood.

TIPS FOR DISCOVERING YOUR VALUE TO OTHERS

→ Remember that you are needed and have gifts that others will benefit from.

→ Keep your eyes open for someone who can use your help.

→ Deliver ample, honest affirmation and encouragement.

→ Keep your listening ears on high alert.

- Be honest about yourself, including your past struggles and paths to redemption.

TIPS FOR TAKING RESPONSIBILITY

- The next time someone gives feedback or constructive criticism, say thank you before saying anything else. It'll build the habit of being open to growth and kill the habit of getting defensive.
- When you apologize or tell someone something that might be uncomfortable, try to imagine what they might be feeling. For example, "I'm sorry for what I did. I can imagine you're probably angry with me right now." It shows the other person that you're trying to understand them. Even if you get it wrong, they'll see that you're trying to connect, and they may well move in your direction.

TIPS FOR BETTER UNDERSTANDING YOUR FATHER OR ROLE MODEL

- Ask your father open-ended questions about his childhood, young adulthood, and his career. How did he struggle? How does he still struggle today? What were his happiest times? What are his fears—past and present?
- Ask your father for his advice on the challenges you face. Share the fears and emotions you have when it comes to decisions you need to make and seek his input and wisdom. If you take his advice, be sure to express your gratitude to him.

- Expand the role of a father figure in your life beyond your own father. Seek out multiple role models or mentors who are older and have developed resilience to get through life's challenges. Make a point to connect with a father figure at least once a month, whether you're talking with someone you know well or beginning to explore with someone new.
- Don't fear faith but be open to exploring with curiosity.

TIPS FOR STANDING UP FOR YOURSELF

- Ask yourself, *Do I give others constant praise, even when I'm not being authentic? Do I say yes to everything, even if I find myself frequently wanting out? Do I feel guilty if I can't fulfill someone else's request? Do I consistently neglect my personal needs and boundaries?*
- The next time you find yourself in a situation where you're tempted to avoid conflict and give in to your fawning response, pause for five seconds instead of answering immediately and ask yourself, *What would it look like for me to stand strong in a loving way in this situation?*
- If you feel frustrated by close relationships, including those with a girlfriend, spouse, or parents, think about what specifically bothers you and approach them using the word *I* so you are speaking for yourself.
- Work at setting boundaries. If you feel overworked and tired, set hours and decline after-work invitations. If you feel your partner isn't on the same page, express needs and expectations clearly. If you feel you are being taken advantage of, establish terms and share them clearly.

- Take a deep breath when you feel bothered or threatened by the different views and opinions of others. Remember that you grow stronger by listening and learning.

TIPS FOR ASSASSINATING ANXIETY

- When anxiety strikes, try this belly-breathing technique: Place your hand on your stomach and inhale deeply so see your hand rise like a balloon. Do this breathing slowly in and out for sixty seconds as your anxiety deflates.
- Ask yourself, *What am I afraid of? How is my anxiety trying to get my attention? How can I address it?*
- Write down the fears and your feelings about the root causes, list strengths you can use to combat them, and generate coping strategies that can help you find relief from anxiety.

TIPS FOR MAKING MONEY WORK FOR YOU

- Remember, money won't make you a man, and money alone won't bring you joy. When you are pursuing a financial or material goal like a new car or house, ask yourself, *What do I really want?* It's probably not the thing itself, but rather what that thing can bring you. Understanding the root of your desire helps you determine whether or not to pursue it.
- Cultivating financial discipline in your twenties and thirties can help you achieve your goals. Invest and give, and you will get in return.

- → Building wealth and financial strength slowly and consistently over time is always the best strategy. Get-rich-quick schemes are enticing but all too often result in failure.
- → Take a step back and think about what you can value above and beyond the endless pursuit of things.

TIPS FOR STAYING GROUNDED WITH SEX

- → Talk out loud with someone you trust about the issues relating to sex. When we keep our feelings about sex in the dark, we are setting ourselves up to feeling stuck.
- → Ask yourself, *What benefit am I getting from hooking up besides feeling good in the moment?*
- → Ask yourself, *How might I feel after a hookup, and how might the other person feel?* (It will impact them too, even if they are consenting to it and want it.)
- → Visualize the marriage you want. Then do some reverse engineering to see what it'll take to achieve that.
- → What's your take on this question? *Will hookups push me closer to or farther from my goals regarding marriage?*

TIPS FOR CHANGING YOUR BODY AND CHANGING YOUR BRAIN

- → Commit to one easy habit you can consistently carry out, such as going to the gym with a fitness plan or establishing a regular pattern of running or biking. If you're already working out, add something new to keep it interesting.

- → Set achievable goals, say them out loud to yourself and someone else, and celebrate milestones in victory.
- → Find friends or a community to engage with, celebrate their achievements, and listen to their challenges.
- → Remember that you are positively shaping both your mind and your body. During workouts, embrace thoughts about your life as you currently experience it, your work, and your family and how you can be stronger in all of these aspects.

TIPS FOR LEARNING DISCIPLINE

- Think about the characteristics you admire in a strong and well-respected man and imagine yourself having those characteristics.
- Spend quiet time envisioning yourself in the future as your best self. Imagine or draw a literal map that plots the way to get there. Revise your migration map as needed along the way.
- Practice strengthening your discipline by setting specific, achievable goals and giving yourself strong noes and yeses in response as needed to stick to the goals.

TIPS FOR FINDING YOUR PURPOSE

- Think about the legacy you want to leave, the difference you want to make through your life. Ask yourself,

What do I want my life to count for? How do I want people to remember me?

- Begin now to shape your life around the purpose that is growing within you. Even when hardships come, stay focused on the character you are committed to building and the impact for good that you want to make.

NOTES

CHAPTER 1: YOU ARE NOT A PUPPET (TAKE ACTION TO KILL DISTRACTION)

1. Jon Gordon, *The Energy Bus* (Wiley, 2007), 41, 47, 164.
2. Christian Montag et al., "Problematic Social Media Use in Childhood and Adolescence, *Addictive Behaviors* 153 (2024), www.sciencedirect.com /science/article/pii/S0306460324000297.
3. Brian N. Chin, "Why Social Media Screen Time Is So Bad for Sleep?" *Scientific American*, April 9, 2025, www.scientificamerican.com/article /why-social-media-screen-time-is-so-bad-for-sleep/.
4. Naveen Kumar, "Average Time Spent on Social Media Per Day (2025 Statistics)," Demandsage, June 19, 2025, www.demandsage.com /average-time-spent-on-social-media/.
5. Justin Zorn and Leigh Marz, "The Busier You Are, the More You Need Quiet Time," *Harvard Business Review*, March 17, 2017, https://hbr .org/2017/03/the-busier-you-are-the-more-you-need-quiet-time.

CHAPTER 2: RUN THROUGH DISCOMFORT

1. Kaitlin Woolley and Ayelet Fishbach, "Motivating Personal Growth by Seeking Discomfort," *Psychological Science* 33, no. 4 (2022): 510–23, www.researchgate.net/publication/359590301_Motivating_Personal _Growth_by_Seeking_Discomfort.
2. U.S. Department of Homeland Security, "Human Trafficking Quick Facts," accessed August 4, 2025, www.dhs.gov /human-trafficking-quick-facts.

3. Wayne Parry, "Poll Shows Young Men in the US Are More at Risk for Gambling Addiction Than the General Population," Associated Press, September 20, 2024, https://apnews.com/article/sports-betting-compulsive-gambling-addiction-d4d0b7a8465e5be0b451b115cab0fb15.
4. Woolley and Fishbach, "Motivating Personal Growth."

CHAPTER 3: FIND YOUR INJURIES

1. J. Douglas Bremner, "Traumatic Stress: Effects on the Brain," *Dialogues in Clinical Neuroscience* 8, no. 4 (2006): 445–61, www.tandfonline.com/doi/full/10.31887/DCNS.2006.8.4/jbremner.
2. "Understanding Child Trauma," Substance Abuse and Mental Health Services Administration (SAMHSA), accessed July 25, 2025, https://library.samhsa.gov/sites/default/files/sma16-4923_0.pdf.
3. Erin C. Dunn et al., "Developmental Timing of Trauma Exposure and Emotion Dysregulation in Adulthood: Are There Sensitive Periods When Trauma Is Most Harmful?" *Journal of Affective Disorders* 227 (2018): 869–77, https://pmc.ncbi.nlm.nih.gov/articles/PMC5805641/.
4. Louise Langman and Man Cheung Chung, "The Relationship Between Forgiveness, Spirituality, Traumatic Guilt and Posttraumatic Stress Disorder (PTSD) Among People with Addiction," *Psychiatry Quarterly* 84, no. 1 (2013): 11–26, https://pubmed.ncbi.nlm.nih.gov/22585109/.
5. "About Adverse Childhood Experiences," US Centers for Disease Control, October 8, 2024, www.cdc.gov/aces/about/index.html.

CHAPTER 4: DRAFT YOUR TEAM

1. Quoted in Darren Hardy, *The Compound Effect: Jumpstart Your Income, Your Life, Your Success* (Vanguard, 2010), 127.
2. Françoise Côté, Gaston Godin, and Camille Gagné, "Identification of Factors Promoting Abstinence from Smoking in a Cohort of Elementary Schoolchildren," *Preventive Medicine* 39, no. 4 (2004): 695–703, www.sciencedirect.com/science/article/abs/pii/S0091743504001227.
3. James Niels Rosenquist, James H. Fowler, and Nicholas A. Christakis, "Social Network Determinants of Depression," *Molecular Psychiatry* 16, no. 3 (2011): 273–81, https://pubmed.ncbi.nlm.nih.gov/20231839/;

Nicholas A. Christakis and James H. Fowler, "The Collective Dynamics of Smoking in a Large Social Network," *New England Journal of Medicine* 358, no. 21 (2008): 2249–58, https://pubmed.ncbi.nlm.nih.gov/18499567/; Nicholas A. Christakis and James H. Fowler, " The Spread of Obesity in a Large Social Network over 32 Years," *New England Journal of Medicine* 357, no. 4 (2007): 370–79, https://pubmed.ncbi.nlm.nih.gov/17652652/.

4. Declan Fitzpatrick, "The Power of Social Conformity," Achology, accessed July 28, 2025, https://achology.com/psychology/social-conformity-insights-from-the-asch-conformity-experiment/.
5. Neal M. Malamuth, Tamara Addison, and Mary Koss, "Pornography and Sexual Aggression: Are There Reliable Effects and Can We Understand Them?" *Annual Review of Sex Research* 11, no. 1 (2000): 26–91, www.researchgate.net/publication/11985517_Pornography_and_sexual_aggression_Are_there_reliable_effects_and_can_we_understand_them.
6. Jim Collins. "First Who, Then What," JimCollins.com, accessed August 4, 2025, www.jimcollins.com/concepts/first-who-then-what.html.
7. Jon Gordon, *The Energy Bus: 10 Rules to Fuel Your Life, Work, and Team with Positive Energy* (Wiley, 2007), 22.
8. Keith McFarland, *The Breakthrough Company* (Crown Business, 2008), 168.
9. Elliot T. Berkman, "The Neuroscience of Goals and Behavior Change," *Consulting Psychology Journal* 70, no. 1 (2018): 28–44, www.researchgate.net/publication/318542415_The_Neuroscience_of_Goals_and_Behavior_Change.

CHAPTER 5: ASK YOURSELF WHY

1. Monica Diana Olteanu, "Female Brain Versus Male Brain," NeuroRelay, October 7, 2012, https://neurorelay.com/2012/10/07/female-brain-versus-male-brain/.
2. George F. Koob and Michel Le Moal, "Plasticity of Reward Neurocircuitry and the 'Dark Side' of Drug Addiction," *Nature Neuroscience* 8, no. 11 (2005): 1442–44, https://www.researchgate.net/publication/7514760_Plasticity_of_reward_neurocircuitry_and_the_'dark_side'_of_drug_addiction.

3. Simon Sinek, *Start with Why: How Great Leaders Inspire Everyone to Take Action* (Portfolio/Penguin, 2009).
4. Beth Greenfield, "The 'Triple Threat' Endangering Worker Well-Being and Undermining Productivity—Especially for Gen Z," *Fortune Well*, June 18, 2025, https://fortune.com/well/2025/06/18/american-workers-gen-z-triple-threat-undermining-productivity/.

CHAPTER 6: THE SECRET OF THE CAVEMAN

1. Dallas Willard, *Renovation of the Heart: Putting on the Character of Christ*, rev. ed. (NavPress, 2021), 125.
2. Laura Upenieks, "Unpacking the Relationship Between Prayer and Anxiety: A Consideration of Prayer Types and Expectations in the United States," *Journal of Religion and Health* 62, no. 3 (2023): 1810–31, https://pubmed.ncbi.nlm.nih.gov/36449251/.

CHAPTER 7: CAN'T DO WITHOUT YOU

1. Adrian Gostick, "Harvard Research Reveals the #1 Key to Living Longer and Happier," *Forbes*, August 15, 2023, www.forbes.com/sites/adriangostick/2023/08/15/harvard-research-reveals-the-1-key-to-living-longer-and-happier/.
2. Cited in John C. Maxwell, *25 Ways to Win with People: How to Make Others Feel Like a Million Bucks* (Thomas Nelson, 2005), 89.

CHAPTER 8: THAT'S ON ME

1. Dick Dodds and Donna Swiniarski, *The First 120 Minutes: A Guide to Crisis Management in Education* (Canadian Education Association, 1994), 9–16.
2. John Macon Gillespie, "Ole Miss' Jaxson Dart Focused on Finishing Season 'The Right Way' After Florida Loss," *Sports Illustrated*, November 23, 2024, www.si.com/college/olemiss/football/ole-miss-jaxson-dart-focused-on-finishing-season-the-right-way-after-florida-loss-01jdd5p46q57.
3. David Rosenberg, "Florida Football Time Machine: Tebow Delivers 'The Promise' Speech," *USA Today*, September 27, 2022, https://gatorswire

.usatoday.com/story/sports/college/gators/football/2022/09/27/florida-football-tim-tebow-the-promise/78637524007/.

CHAPTER 9: YOUR FATHER (OR FATHER FIGURE) ISN'T PERFECT

1. David P. Farrington et al., "The Concentration of Offenders in Families, and Family Criminality in the Prediction of Boys' Delinquency," *Journal of Adolescence* 24, no. 5 (2001): 579–96, https://pubmed.ncbi.nlm.nih.gov/11676506/.
2. David P. Farrington, Geoffrey C. Barnes, and Sandra Lambert, "The Concentration of Offending in Families," *Legal and Criminological Psychology* 1, no. 1 (1996): 47–63, https://bpspsychub.onlinelibrary.wiley.com/doi/abs/10.1111/j.2044-8333.1996.tb00306.x.
3. National Institute on Drug Abuse (NIDA), *Addiction and Health*, last modified July 6, 2020, https://nida.nih.gov/publications/drugs-brains-behavior-science-addiction/addiction-health.
4. Luca Rollè et al., "Father Involvement and Cognitive Development in Early and Middle Childhood: A Systematic Review," *Frontiers in Psychology* 10, no. 2405 (2019), https://pmc.ncbi.nlm.nih.gov/articles/PMC6823210/.
5. "Dietary Guidelines for Americans: 2020–2025," 9th ed., U.S. Department of Agriculture and U.S. Department of Health and Human Services, December 2020, accessed August 4, 2025, www.dietaryguidelines.gov/sites/default/files/2021-03/Dietary_Guidelines_for_Americans-2020-2025.pdf.
6. Rachel Minkin, Kim Parker, Juliana Horowitz, and Carolina Aragão, "Parents, Young Adult Children and the Transition to Adulthood," Pew Research Center, January 2024, 35, www.pewresearch.org/wp-content/uploads/sites/20/2024/01/ST_2024.01.25_Parents-Young-Adults_Report.pdf.
7. Minkin et al., "Parents, Young Adult Children and the Transition to Adulthood," 43.
8. Jeff Grabmeier, "Adult Children More Likely to Be Estranged from Dad

Than Mom," Ohio State News, December 15, 2022, https://news.osu.edu/adult-children-more-likely-to-be-estranged-from-dad-than-mom/.

9. Brian J. Grim and Melissa E. Grim, "Belief, Behavior, and Belonging: How Faith Is Indispensable in Preventing and Recovering from Substance Abuse," *Journal of Religious Health* 58, no. 5 (2019): 1713–50, https://pmc.ncbi.nlm.nih.gov/articles/PMC6759672/, italics in original.
10. "Religion's Relationship to Happiness, Civic Engagement and Health Around the World," Pew Research Center, January 31, 2019, www.pewresearch.org/religion/2019/01/31/religions-relationship-to-happiness-civic-engagement-and-health-around-the-world/.
11. T. M. Luhrman, *How God Becomes Real: Kindling the Presence of Invisible Others* (Princeton University Press, 2020), xiv.
12. Gregory A. Smith et al., "Decline of Christianity in the U.S. Has Slowed, May Have Leveled Off," Pew Research Center, February 26, 2025, www.pewresearch.org/religion/2025/02/26/decline-of-christianity-in-the-us-has-slowed-may-have-leveled-off/.
13. Ruth Graham, "In a First Among Christians, Young Men Are More Religious Than Young Women," *New York Times*, September 23, 2024, www.bishop-accountability.org/2024/09/in-a-first-among-christians-young-men-are-more-religious-than-young-women/.
14. W. Bradford Wilcox and Nicholas H. Wolfinger, *Soul Mates: Religion, Sex, Love, and Marriage Among African Americans and Latinos* (Oxford University Press, 2016).

CHAPTER 10: STAND UP FOR YOURSELF

1. "Men Feel Worse About Themselves When Female Partners Succeed, Says New Research," American Psychological Association, August 5, 2013, www.apa.org/news/press/releases/2013/08/men-self-esteem.
2. Pauline Rose Clance, *The Impostor Phenomenon: Overcoming the Fear That Haunts Your Success* (Peachtree, 1985), 9–23.

CHAPTER 11: EMBRACE THE ANXIETY ASSASSIN

1. "American Adults Express Increasing Anxiousness in Annual Poll; Stress and Sleep Are Key Factors Impacting Mental Health," American

Psychiatric Association, May 1, 2024, www.psychiatry.org/news-room/news-releases/annual-poll-adults-express-increasing-anxiousness.

2. Cheryl Strayed, *Brave Enough* (Knopf, 2015), 106.
3. Akira Olsen, "Anxiety Epidemic Among Millennials and Gen Z," Medium, October 10, 2018, https://medium.com/@akiraolsen/anxiety-epidemic-among-millennials-and-gen-z-8f9617ea7a9b.
4. "How Anxiety Impacts Men Versus Women," UNC Men's Health Program, accessed August 4, 2025, www.med.unc.edu/menshealth/how-anxiety-impacts-men-versus-women/.
5. "Men: A Different Depression," American Psychological Association, July 14, 2005, www.apa.org/topics/men-boys/depression.
6. James R. Mahalik, Shaun M. Burns, and Matthew Syzdek, "Masculinity and Perceived Normative Health Behaviors as Predictors of Men's Health Behaviors," *Social Science and Medicine* 64, no. 11 (2007): 2201–9.
7. "*Spider-Man: Homecoming*: Quotes," IMDb, accessed August 4, 2025, www.imdb.com/title/tt2250912/characters/nm0000375/.

CHAPTER 12: MONEY WORKS FOR YOU

1. Sheiresa McRae Ngo, "Most Americans Are Significantly Stressed About Money," *Spokesman-Review*, updated June 14, 2024, www.spokesman.com/stories/2024/jun/12/most-americans-are-significantly-stressed-about-mo/.
2. Lane Gillespie, "Survey: More Than 1 in 4 Americans Feel They Need to Make $150,000 or More to Live Comfortably," Bankrate, June 23, 2025, www.bankrate.com/investing/financial-advisors/financial-freedom-survey/.
3. "Gen Z and Millennials Are Obsessed with the Idea of Being Rich, and It Could Be Leading to Money Dysmorphia," Credit Karma, January 17, 2024, www.creditkarma.com/about/commentary/gen-z-and-millennials-are-obsessed-with-the-idea-of-being-rich-and-it-could-be-leading-to-money-dysmorphia.
4. "Transcript: Tom Brady, Part 3," *60 Minutes*, November 4, 2005, www.cbsnews.com/news/transcript-tom-brady-part-3/.
5. Matthew Ridley et al., "Poverty, Depression, and Anxiety: Causal

Evidence and Mechanisms," *Science* 370 (2020), https://economics.mit.edu/sites/default/files/2022-09/poverty-depression-anxiety-science.pdf.

6. Daniel Kahneman and Angus Deaton, "High Income Improves Evaluation of Life but Not Emotional Well-Being," *Proceedings of the National Academy of Sciences of the United States of America* 107, no. 38 (2010): 16489–93, https://pubmed.ncbi.nlm.nih.gov/20823223/.
7. Suzanne B. O'Brien, "I've Been a Hospice Nurse for 20 Years. People Often Have 4 Confessions on Their Deathbed—Here's What They Teach Us," CNBC, updated March 18, 2025, www.cnbc.com/2025/03/18/hospice-nurse-biggest-regrets-people-have-on-deathbeds-what-it-teaches-us-about-living-happy-meaningful-lives.html.
8. "FDU Poll Finds Online Betting Leads to Problems for Young Men," Fairleigh Dickinson University, September 19, 2024, www.fdu.edu/news/fdu-poll-finds-online-betting-leads-to-problems-for-young-men/.
9. Wyatt Myers, "Is Sports Betting Becoming a Health Problem?," UHealth Collective, September 5, 2024, https://news.umiamihealth.org/en/is-sports-betting-becoming-a-health-problem/.
10. Luke Clark et al., "Gambling Near-Misses Enhance Motivation to Gamble and Recruit Win-Related Brain Circuitry," *Neuron* 61, no. 3 (2009): 481–90, www.cell.com/neuron/fulltext/S0896-6273(09)00037-3; Lauren Rubenstein, "Robinson in *The Conversation*: How Gambling Distorts Reality and Hooks Your Brain," Wesleyan Connection, August 17, 2018, https://newsletter.blogs.wesleyan.edu/2018/08/17/robinson-in-the-conversation-how-gambling-distorts-reality-and-hooks-your-brain/.
11. Jana Arbanas et al., "Earning Trust as AI Takes Hold: 2024 Connected Consumer Survey," Deloitte, December 3, 2024, www.deloitte.com/us/en/insights/industry/telecommunications/connectivity-mobile-trends-survey.html#explore.
12. Jennifer Breheny Wallace, *Never Enough: When Achievement Culture Becomes Toxic—and What We Can Do About It* (Portfolio/Penguin, 2023), xiv.
13. "John D. Rockefeller," New World Encyclopedia, accessed August 4, 2025, www.newworldencyclopedia.org/entry/John_D._Rockefeller.

CHAPTER 13: SEX WON'T SAVE YOU

1. Evan Castillo, "College Students Prefer Finding Relationships Without Dating Apps: Survey," Best Colleges, updated on November 27, 2023, www.bestcolleges.com/news/college-students-dont-love-dating-apps/.
2. Justin R. Garcia et al., "Sexual Hookup Culture: A Review," American Psychological Association, *Review of General Psychology* 16, no. 2 (2012): 161–76, www.apa.org/monitor/2013/02/sexual-hookup-culture.pdf.
3. Maryanne L. Fisher et al., "Feelings of Regret Following Uncommitted Sexual Encounters in Canadian University Students," *Culture, Health and Sexuality* 14, no. 1 (2012): 45–57, https://pubmed.ncbi.nlm.nih.gov/22077716/ https://doi.org/10.1080/13691058.2011.619579.
4. Elizabeth L. Paul, Brian McManus, and Allison Hayes, "'Hookups': Characteristics and Correlates of College Students' Spontaneous and Anonymous Sexual Experiences," *Journal of Sex Research* 37, no. 1 (2000): 76–88, www.tandfonline.com/doi/abs/10.1080/00224490009552023.
5. David G. Blanchflower and Andrew J. Oswald, "Money, Sex, and Happiness: An Empirical Study," National Bureau of Economic Research Working Paper No. 10499 (May 2004), www.nber.org/papers/w10499.
6. Lucy E. Napper et al., "Assessing the Personal Negative Impacts of Hooking Up Experienced by College Students: Gender Differences and Mental Health," *Journal of Sexual Research* 53, no. 7 (2017): 766–75, https://pmc.ncbi.nlm.nih.gov/articles/PMC5184218/.
7. Brian Willoughby et al., "The Myth of Sexual Experience: Why Sexually Inexperienced Dating Couples Actually Go On to Have Stronger Marriages," Wheatley Institute, April 18, 2023, https://wheatley.byu.edu/the-myth-of-sexual-experience.
8. Robyn L. Fielder and Michael P. Carey, "Predictors and Consequences of Sexual 'Hookups' among College Students: A Short-Term Prospective Study," Archives of Sexual Behavior 39, no. 5 (2010): 1105–19, https://pmc.ncbi.nlm.nih.gov/articles/PMC2933280/pdf/nihms223759.pdf.

CHAPTER 14: CHANGE YOUR BODY, CHANGE YOUR BRAIN

1. "Physical Activity Basics: Overcoming Barriers to Physical Activity," CDC, February 5, 2025, www.cdc.gov/physical-activity-basics/overcoming-barriers/index.html.
2. "Exercising to Relax," Harvard Health Report, July 7, 2020, www.health.harvard.edu/staying-healthy/exercising-to-relax.
3. Melanie Radzicki McManus, "Why Exercise Is Also Good for Your Sexual Health," CNN Health, January 29, 2022, www.cnn.com/2022/01/29/health/exercise-good-for-sexual-health-wellness.
4. "Health Risks of an Inactive Style," National Library of Medicine: Medline Plus, accessed August 4, 2025, https://medlineplus.gov/healthrisksofaninactivelifestyle.html.
5. Kathleen Dalton, *Theodore Roosevelt: A Strenuous Life* (Vintage, 2002), 50.
6. Theodore Roosevelt, *The Strenuous Life: Essays and Addresses* (Century, 1902), 2.
7. Quoted in Ansalda Ceba, *The Citizen of a Republic* (Paine and Burgess, 1845), 92.
8. Nazik Elgaddal, Ellen A. Kramarow, and Cynthia Reuben, "Physical Activity Among Adults Aged 18 and Over: United States, 2020," National Center for Health Statistics, NCHS Data Brief no. 443, August 2022, www.cdc.gov/nchs/products/databriefs/db443.htm.
9. "Lane Kiffin: A Storied Path, Journey Coaching Football, Father's Legacy, and QB Jaxson Dart," *Pivot Podcast*, YouTube, April 18, 2025, www.youtube.com/watch?v=RfxlMfj4huk, 30:41.
10. Sammi R. Chekroud et al., "Association Between Physical Exercise and Mental Health in 1.2 Million Individuals in the USA Between 2011 and 2015: A Cross-Sectional Study," *Lancet Psychiatry* 5, no. 9 (2018): 739–46, https://pubmed.ncbi.nlm.nih.gov/30099000/.
11. Jaehyun Joo et al., "The Influence of 15-Week Exercise Training on Dietary Patterns Among Young Adults," *International Journal of Obesity* 43, no. 9 (2019): 1681–90, https://pubmed.ncbi.nlm.nih.gov/30659257/.
12. Christian J. Corral et al., "Physical Activity Frequency Patterns Influence Sleep Architecture in Young Adults," *Journal of Physical Activity*

and Health 22, no. 8 (2025): 1042–50, https://journals.humankinetics.com/view/journals/jpah/22/8/article-p1042.xml.

13. Blake Toppmeyer, "How Greg Sankey's Daily Runs Shaped the SEC's Response to Pandemic," Knox News, updated April 28, 2021, www.knoxnews.com/story/sports/college/university-of-tennessee/football/2021/04/28/greg-sankey-sec-commissioner-running-marathon-southeastern-conference/7375953002/.

CHAPTER 15: DISCIPLINE

1. Nathan Maciborski, "Yankees Magazine: The Road to Immortality," MLB, May 9, 2017, www.mlb.com/news/derek-jeter-s-road-to-immortality-c229214450.
2. Hal E. Hershfield, "Future Self-Continuity: How Conceptions of the Future Self Transform Intertemporal Choice," *Annals of the New York Academy of Sciences* 1235, no. 1 (2011): 30–43, https://pubmed.ncbi.nlm.nih.gov/22023566/.
3. Heather S. Lonczak, "40+ Benefits of Self-Control and Self-Discipline," Positive Psychology, June 19, 2019, https://positivepsychology.com/benefits-self-control-discipline/.

CHAPTER 16: HONED, CULTIVATED, AND FORGED

1. The story is adapted from Loren Eiseley, "The Star Thrower," in *The Unexpected Universe* (Harcourt, Brace and World, 1969).
2. Patrick L. Hill and Nicholas A. Turiano, "Purpose in Life as a Predictor of Mortality Across Adulthood," *Psychological Science* 25, no. 7 (2014): 1482–86, https://pubmed.ncbi.nlm.nih.gov/24815612/.
3. "About Us: Our History," Celebrate Recovery, accessed August 4, 2025, https://celebraterecovery.com/about/.

From the Publisher

GREAT BOOKS

ARE EVEN BETTER WHEN THEY'RE SHARED!

Help other readers find this one:

- Post a review at your favorite online bookseller
- Post a picture on a social media account and share why you enjoyed it
- Send a note to a friend who would also love it—or better yet, give them a copy

Thanks for reading!